Dyslexia Unravelled

Rita Treacy

ABOUT THE AUTHOR

Rita Treacy graduated from Trinity College Dublin in 1986 with a BSc (Hons) degree in Remedial Linguistics, after discovering in her first year that she had dyslexia. Following one year of work experience in a community care clinic in Dublin, she relocated to Australia where she specialised in specific learning difficulties/dyslexia and associated language difficulties in children and adolescents.

She returned to Ireland in 1991 and worked for twelve years, in a multidisciplinary team, in the St John of God Lucena Clinic, Child and Adolescent Mental Health Services (CAMHS), becoming principal speech and language therapist and head of department.

In 2002, Rita established her own full-time private practice to further her specialism in the area. During that time she developed an online programme called WordsWorthLearning specifically to help children and young people overcome their reading and spelling difficulties.

DYSLEXIA UNRAVELLED

An Irish Guide to a Global Problem

Rita Treacy

Edited by Dr Marie Murray

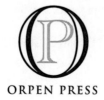

ORPEN PRESS

Published by
Orpen Press
Upper Floor, Unit K9
Greenogue Business Park
Rathcoole
Co. Dublin
Ireland
email: info@orpenpress.com
www.orpenpress.com

Paperback ISBN 978-1-78605-025-0
ePub ISBN 978-1-78605-026-7
Kindle ISBN 978-1-78605-027-4
PDF ISBN 978-1-78605-028-1

Printed in Dublin by SPRINTprint Ltd

To my parents, Pat and Eileen,
for their unwavering love and support.

Acknowledgements

I would like to thank Dr Marie Murray, clinical psychologist, for convincing me that I could take on and complete this massive task and for the immense support, guidance and wisdom that she provided throughout the process.

A note of gratitude also to all the parents and children I have worked with over the last 30 years, whose stories and experiences have been the backbone to this book.

My thanks also to Orpen Press, particularly Eileen O'Brien and Gerry Kelly, for their support and professionalism at every step of the way throughout this process.

My sincerest thanks to my brother Pat, his wife, Linda, and their four children for their unfailing support.

Of course, the task was made easier with the enormous loving support, encouragement and patience of my husband, David.

FOREWORD

Dyslexia, like many complex conditions, is visible if you know how to spot it. There are clues from the earliest developmental stage. Yet too often its signals go unnoticed or misinterpreted and of course the longer it takes for accurate diagnosis the greater the misery it inflicts.

Research shows that the consequences of delay are academic, behavioural, social and psychological. But these are abstract terms that do not describe the daily lived emotional experiences of a child who struggles to read; a child who feels different to other children; a child who dreads each school day; a child who just wants to be the same as the other children in school. Dyslexia unidentified can leave children, adolescents and the adults they become feeling not just academically inept but personally humiliated, vocationally compromised, professionally thwarted, socially undermined and psychologically distressed.

And if this sounds extreme, then speech and language therapist Rita Treacy, the author of this book, shows just how deeply being dyslexic can eat into the mind, the heart, the self-esteem, the confidence and the identity of sufferers. Those early childhood experiences and adolescent agonies etch themselves on a person in ways that only those who are dyslexic can truly understand.

It is this personal story that Rita Treacy brings to her professional work that makes this book unique. Growing up with dyslexia and turning that initial disadvantage into a quest to ensure that others would not suffer as she did, Rita understands dyslexia from every perspective, and her years of study, of research, of assessment, of clinical practice, of programme development and of multidisciplinary collaboration shine through every chapter in this important book. No parent need fear that they will miss the early markers of dyslexia nor that they will be left without the support they need to understand what to do at every stage along the way. From the initial query, through assessment to secure diagnosis followed by successful interventions, everything a parent or professional needs to know about dyslexia is provided comprehensively in this book.

Dyslexia Unravelled gives information on the multidisciplinary nature of assessments, and the terminology associated with standardised tests administered by psychologists, teachers, speech and language therapists, occupational therapists and all who interact professionally with the 'dyslexic' child. The book provides appreciation of the difference between dyslexia and other reading/spelling disorders in a way that no other book does, unravelling these complex clinical similarities and difficulties so clearly for the reader. The book explains how, why, when and from whom to seek help; the emotional impact of diagnosis; and the dangers of undiagnosed dyslexia or incorrect, inadequate intervention, especially for those who give up and drop out of school. In this era of assistive technology, Rita recognises the educational implications of dyslexia for those babies who may hold a smartphone before they ever see a book and what resources, agencies, grants, supports and services are available because swift diagnosis and effective intervention are so important for mental health and happiness too.

Shining her personal and professional light on dyslexia, Rita Treacy knows what she calls 'the acute anxiety, shame and embarrassment' of being dyslexic; she knows how it feels to be intelligent and think that you are 'stupid'; to work hard and be considered 'lazy'; to live a life of coping, camouflage and cover-up, carrying the hurt of 'difference' into secondary school; the challenges of dyslexia into exams; and the trials of third-level academic and clinical life with dyslexia. More importantly, Rita knows – and demonstrates by writing this wonderful book – how what initially seems to be a dark disadvantage can unearth undreamt of talents, how grappling with a specific learning difficulty can uncover creative abilities that might not otherwise appear, how apparent disadvantage can become an asset, and how one person's affliction may become an instrument to assist many people in their lives. History is replete with those now-famous creators, writers, scientists and inventors whose dyslexia and different learning styles ignited ingenious creativity for the benefit of all.

Rita Treacy's own wish for this book is that it will reassure anyone who is discouraged by academic difference to know that they have talent and to find it and to understand that intelligence is what you do with your abilities however different or diverse the learning paths may be.

Literacy is liberation. We live in a world of words. Despite how extensively technology may bypass the need to read quickly, write legibly, spell accurately or convey ideas in written form, reading and writing – or 'reeling and writhing' to quote Lewis Carroll's *Alice's Adventures in Wonderland* – remain the keys that unlock the mysteries of learning and educational life. *Dyslexia Unravelled* takes those keys, unlatches dyslexia and opens wide the door to diverse ways of learning. It is my great privilege to commend and recommend this book.

Dr Marie Murray, editor and clinical psychologist, PhD, M.Psych. Sc., BA (Hons Psych.), C. Psychol. PsSI, Reg. FTAI

CONTENTS

BEING DYSLEXIC:
THE HUMILIATION OF BEING DIFFERENT

This book tells two interwoven stories: a personal story, which discusses my own experience of growing up with dyslexia; and a professional story, which summaries how I started a professional project to help others. My personal story explores the emotional, educational and psychological factors of growing up with dyslexia, especially before my diagnosis. My professional story is about how, by becoming a speech and language therapist and by specialising in the subject of literacy and dyslexia, I have converted the burden of dyslexia into a gift both for myself and for others, which I am now setting out to share with you.

I wish that when I was a child someone knew what I now know: exactly what dyslexia is; how to spot it, understand it, accommodate it and manage it; and how to intervene educationally so that it need not cause the distress and embarrassment I experienced before it was identified in me. To this day, I remember vividly when I was eventually identified – in my late teens – as having classic dyslexia. Dyslexia is defined as:

> ... a continuum of specific learning difficulties related to the acquisition of basic skills in reading, spelling and/or writing, such difficulties being unexplained in relation to

an individual's other abilities and educational experiences. Dyslexia can be described at the neurological, cognitive and behavioural levels. It is typically characterised by inefficient information processing, including difficulties in phonological processing, working memory, rapid naming and automaticity of basic skills. Difficulties in organisation, sequencing and motor skills may also be present.[1]

To discover at that stage in my life that the difficulties I had encountered all my school years had a name, 'dyslexia', caused me both comfort and distress in equal measure. It was of course comforting to have it finally acknowledged that I was neither stupid nor lazy (adjectives assigned to me at intervals at school) but that I simply needed to learn differently. Yet, I also felt acute anxiety, shame and embarrassment at the diagnosis because I had spent so many years feeling different and here my difference was confirmed. In the early 1980s, dyslexia was not a badge I wore openly because there were so many negative connotations associated with the condition, unfortunately some of which still exist today. I hope this book will dispel any remaining connotations and reveal dyslexia for the extraordinary paradox it is, additionally revealing the strange benefits or strengths it can bring to those who live with it.

Learning differently should not cause embarrassment. Education should not focus on defining deficit but should appreciate diversity in learning styles, differences in perception, variations in interpretations and individuality of expression. The reality of multiple forms of intelligence should be a cause for celebration of human intellectual diversity and it is time to stop working just to the norm but valuing those who march to a different drum. The beat some hear, that others do not, has historically often brought revelations and dimensions to thinking that has only occurred with difference.

Once I learned to understand myself in this way, dyslexia changed from a burden I carried to a gift I could manipulate to help others, because I could understand at the deepest level what being dyslexic meant. Experiencing it, learning about it, studying it professionally, and developing programmes to help those who have it has been an odyssey of epic proportions. However, now there are many discoveries made, tales to be told, information to be given, perspectives to be shared and, most of all, reassurance for everyone who is dyslexic. They can achieve what may seem to be the impossible.

But the story to be told is not just a personal story of my dyslexia. This book draws from the rich information gleaned from thousands of people I have met and assessed, from their individual case histories I've taken at the assessment and interview stage with the parents of my students who have a specific learning difficulty and from the insights I have gained from those students too. I want to share all that I have gained from these interviews and from working with and treating the problem with each of these students because, while each person is unique, there are common patterns that emerge in how dyslexia expresses itself in each individual. The commonality of these patterns offers intriguing and enlightening perspectives on this worldwide literacy issue. For example, for many years I was perplexed, as were my family, as to the cause of my difficulties. Yet the signs and symptoms of classic dyslexia were visible in everything I did. However, no one clearly identified them or understood their significance. My parents often recount affectionate anecdotes about the things I did as an infant and child, oblivious to all signals of a learning difficulty in my developmental history. One particular story is that I 'bum-shuffled', at speed, until I was 22 months old, a sign of possible future dyslexia. Even today I can at times be physically inept or clumsy, because my motor skills can still present challenges, often in the most unexpected places. I was also a very quiet child, so much so that my father, in his father-of-the-bride speech at my wedding, announced that I spent a lot of my time 'in my own little world'; and he is right, I did. To a point this is still true today and I cherish those daydreaming moments, because sometimes in these 'switched off' periods a literacy puzzle that may have been bothering me for a while suddenly becomes clearer. That is how ideas germinate. That is how dreams are made. There is often more happening in the head of the dreamer than people realise. Ironically, the same sort of dreaming happened while I was in the throes of developing my WordsWorthLearning programme for remediating reading and spelling problems. I would often get clarity on something in the middle of the night and eventually I had to set up a whiteboard outside my bedroom so that I could get up and jot down my inspiration quickly, in my sleepy haze, before it disappeared back into the recesses of my mind.

In the course of my work as a speech and language therapist and literacy consultant I would regularly hear parents and teachers describe a student in question as 'a daydreamer'. I now realise this is not necessarily a negative trait. I believe that from dreams emerge wondrous imaginative creations and vision. If we close off dreaming, we close off imagination. If we close off imagination, we may shut down creativity and in so doing obstruct developments that would occur if we would just let the dreamers dream them.

Although I was never assessed for a language difficulty, I know anecdotally, and now understand professionally as a speech and language therapist, that I mispronounced words as a child. This was not from an articulation perspective but from an inadequate awareness of syllabication or sound sequences. I am still, as an adult, prone to the odd malapropism, mixed metaphor or mispronunciation, as anyone who may have heard my hour-long radio interview with the late Gerry Ryan on my own dyslexia and subsequent work in the field might have noticed, especially my frequent mispronunciation of the word 'etcetera'. Indeed, times of pressure and stress can still bring about funny ways of expressing myself, which I have learned now to value and enjoy rather than allow anyone to embarrass me about them.

While I am not necessarily artistic, I *am* creative and, despite my fine motor skills letting me down at times, I love to make things, which began at a very young age. I have a fond memory of – having mastered Mum's Singer sewing machine – deciding to sew the sheets from my sister's bed together to make a large whale for my younger brother to play with. My mother was none too pleased, particularly as a lot of her soft furnishings disappeared into the filling. Nevertheless, it has also been this creative streak which has inspired the development of my reading and spelling programme. Creativity has not only remediated my own literacy problems, but has also helped thousands of my students with their reading and spelling difficulties.

A high percentage of students I see in private practice today are artistic and creative and a large part of their identity comes from their strengths in this visual domain. This is an area I believe is not given enough status or importance in education today. Creativity is essential in our developing world and it is no coincidence that NASA employs many dyslexic staff because it needs creative people who can think outside the box. It is well known that many successful entrepreneurs have dyslexia, for example, Sir Richard Branson, founder of Virgin Group; Steve Jobs, founder of Apple Inc.; and Bill Gates, founder of Microsoft. Several of these and other brilliant entrepreneurs failed within the one-system-fits-all traditional educational approach to teaching literacy. It was their creativity that provided the impetus to go on to achieve greater things.

I am the middle child of five children and my siblings were all high academic achievers. I was not. You can imagine how different that made me feel. I have early memories from day one in school, struggling to learn sequences such as the alphabet, tables, rhymes and poems. To this day, I still have difficulty with my times tables, learning to recite poems or accurately remembering the lyrics of songs. My solution has always been 'if in doubt make up your own' – now there is creativity!

In second class at primary school, the teacher, a kind nun of advanced years called Sister Malachy, knew I was having difficulties and took me under her wing. She would do extra reading and maths with me during the morning break time. In the mid-1960s there were special classes for children with special needs, such as intellectual disability, but not for children who were deemed bright but underachieving. In hindsight, Sr Malachy's help was much appreciated and kindly given, but of course it added to my distress and anxiety at the time because I could see my friends playing in the playground outside while I was working. There was I getting extra lessons because I was different, mindful that my friends knew only too well why I was inside and not outside playing with them, which maybe is a metaphor for what happens to you if you are dyslexic at school.

Although selectively parents and students can be offered additional learning support in school for problematic subjects, this is often at the expense of a subject the student is good at or even excels in, on the basis that the weak area needs attention. Depriving someone of the experience of achieving and enjoying their strengths to remediate their difficulties is a double-edged sword. The subjects those with dyslexia are good at often include creative activities such as art classes or project work, which are important for self-expression. When you have a specific learning difficulty your self-esteem suffers greatly, so it is important that students with dyslexia do not lose out on their strong subject. Being deprived of the boost of enjoying their strong subject diminishes further their already damaged self-esteem. In fact, every effort should be made to retain the subjects or activities where the dyslexic student can gain recognition and affirmation of their talents and not have them clash with learning support time, otherwise resentment about help can build up if it is at the expense of spending time positively at school.

Following my primary education, my distress was further compounded when I had to leave home at twelve years of age to become a boarder and attend a secondary Gaelscoil. My older sisters had attended the school before me without any difficulty, so it was assumed that this setting would suit me too. It didn't of course, but there was no 'out' to be considered; it was a case of you must work harder. Tragically, Irish remains a total mystery to me, perhaps because it was a source of huge anxiety and stress when I was young. I believe Gaelscoileanna are superb educational settings, but only if you have a facility for languages and are not struggling with either a language difficulty or a specific learning difficulty as they create a double disadvantage. Oddly enough, I managed to camouflage my literacy difficulties quite well and achieved an average standard because I had begun to develop my own memory aids – using mind-map-like structures to summarise chapters – much to the confusion of my classmates. It was only much later, when I was working in Australia, that I discovered mind mapping and I continue to be a huge advocator of Tony Buzan's mind-mapping strategies, utilising the techniques in my own day-to-day work, planning and presentations.

Luckily, I had a good group of friends at school and without ever actually discussing my difficulties they recognised them. They sometimes helped me when I was called upon to read aloud in Irish. They would whisper troublesome words to me to help me through the ordeal. I still have anxiety dreams about reading aloud in a language that makes no sense to me. Today the vast majority of students I see in private practice, particularly those showing classic dyslexia, really struggle with the literacy component of the Irish language. Whereas I acknowledge Irish is a beautiful, descriptive language, it is also a bizarre language in terms of spelling structure. My Scottish husband sometimes brings to my attention the spellings on road signposts, for example it baffles him how one would get the pronunciation 'Leery' from 'Laoghaire', and I can only agree. I suppose travelling through Wales might put it all in perspective; who can pronounce 'Llanfairpwllgwyngyllgogerychwyrndrobwllllantysiliogogogoch'? It is interesting that many students who experience a significant difficulty learning Irish do not necessarily experience a difficulty to the same extent learning other languages such as French, Spanish or German. This may be because there is a more logical sound–symbol association and rule structure in those languages that is not too dissimilar to English. This is something that needs to be given more consideration when evaluating a student's eligibility for an Irish language exemption from their curriculum.

Recognising early signs is critical for early identification of a specific learning difficulty. On reaching the glorious milestone of 50 years of age, I decided to try to find out more about my own beginning. With my parents' permission I wrote to the hospital I was born in and asked for a copy of my birth records. Realistically I didn't expect them to be available but a copy of the original document promptly arrived in the post. After reading the single page, my husband jokingly announced that I must have been the inspiration for the blockbuster movie *Avatar*. The birth notes read 'infant – blue all over – given O_2'. I discussed this with my parents and neither, to their memory, was aware this had occurred or that it could have a negative impact on my development. Interestingly, in January 2014 Eilish O'Regan, health correspondent with the *Irish Independent*, reported on a study being carried out in University College Cork. The study, being conducted by Professor Geraldine Boylan and Dr Deirdre Murray, looked at newborns who had experienced a lack of oxygen around the time of birth, otherwise known as hypoxic-ischemic encephalopathy (HIE). The study revealed that 18–20 per cent of newborns who experienced even mild HIE at birth had 'learning or behavioural difficulties at five years, including speech delay, autism, attention deficit disorder and dyspraxia'. In addition, they were found to have 'decreased processing speeds and poor working memory'.[2] As this is such an interesting topic I will discuss it in more detail in Chapter 2.

Finding out about my birth details was a eureka moment for me – after years of doubt and shame about being the academic black sheep of the family, I felt I had discovered the probable cause of my dyslexia. It clearly wasn't genetic or familial.

Because of my need to find out what had happened to make me different I understand why all the parents I interview ask me the same four questions I have asked myself:

- What is the problem?
- Why does my child/do I have this problem?
- Could it have been prevented?
- Can it be cured?

As a speech and language therapist, while protecting client confidentiality, I can and do ask probing questions during the assessment process to research all the factors and patterns that could give us more insight into dyslexia. My interviews with parents include gathering personal information regarding pregnancy, the child's birth and developmental details, and the family history. Access to this information helps me to make a differential diagnosis; that is, in this case, to weigh up and decide between dyslexia and a reading/spelling delay or disorder. Years of experience have led me to believe that these conditions are not synonymous and that they require different remedial therapy paths. Accurate diagnosis is imperative to manage expectations; I am only too aware that dyslexia is a lifelong condition that manifests itself in many ways with complicated associated difficulties; these too change in how they are shown over time. These difficulties can present themselves primarily in the auditory, visual, motor or language domains and these will be explored in detail in Chapters 2–5.

As someone who is dyslexic, but is now consciously competent at reading and spelling, I have not only come to terms with my life as a person with dyslexia but now I truly do appreciate, enjoy and embrace my dyslexia for the insights it has given me. I always tell clients about my own dyslexia at the time of assessment so they will know that I truly understand all their fears, worries and concerns. This fosters unique trust and knowing between the parent, student and myself. Parents are more comfortable divulging in-depth personal and familial information with me because they know I understand and this in turn contributes to the success of the interventions that I suggest and implement. It is this collected and collated anonymous information that provides the content for this book; no identifying information or stories are told. But with the amalgam of the assessment interviews I have conducted over the years I have acquired understanding of the eight common factors in dyslexia, which I will discuss in the chapters of this book in the following way:

Chapter 2 – What to Look Out For: Early Signs that Might Signal a Later Problem

This chapter is designed to tell you about the early signs that may alert you to a problem or that might indicate an existing literacy difficulty or the probability of a difficulty emerging at a later stage. Identifying a difficulty early can save years of strife and failure.

Chapter 3 – Trusting Your Gut Instinct: When to Look for Help

Parents need to be encouraged to trust their gut instinct if they feel their child is underperforming or may have a literacy difficulty. If nothing is being done about it in school, contact the school and talk to the teacher. Don't be content with reassurance that your child will grow out of it because that is too big a chance to take. In my clinical experience, children often don't grow out of it; and as a result they can end up falling even further behind. This chapter will help you to understand what to do and why you should act quickly.

Chapter 4 – Understanding Assessments

Parents need to understand the multidisciplinary nature of the assessment process and the hierarchy or order of the assessments their child may need to undergo; in other words, which professionals to approach and in what order. This can vary according to the age and ability of the student. Many parents get confused when they receive a report from school or a professional that they don't fully understand, especially if the report contains a lot of unfamiliar professional jargon or gives test scores and other information that parents do not know how to interpret. Unfortunately, there is a danger that something can be missed; or the wrong course of action taken; or worse still, no action at all taken because of the bewildering range of recommendations made. This chapter will guide you and help you to ensure that you know the logic behind the assessment process and what the reports mean.

Chapter 5 – When Is Dyslexia Not Dyslexia

The complex classification of a specific learning difficulty is explained in this chapter using a three-tier classification, which explains the difference between dyslexia and a reading/spelling disorder, based on my professional experience. It also explores the impact that can arise from a misdiagnosis in terms of treatment and it discusses the positive and negative effects of using the dyslexia label.

Chapter 6 – Choosing the Right Help

In today's educational world there is a plethora of materials and interventions available, many incorrectly presenting themselves as the panacea for all ills. Many parents report that they are confused by this, particularly when a professional report recommends a number of interventions that could be used to remediate a problem, some of which actually utilise conflicting teaching methods. Parents want guidance on what to use and what to avoid, based on professional independent research; this chapter sets out to assist them in this.

Chapter 7 – Working Together: Home, School and Others

Parents constantly talk about how much they need a more collaborative approach between the school and teacher and the student and parent; this also includes other associated professionals. A significant number of parents with a child attending learning support have no idea what is being done during the support sessions and this can cause concern for them. Greater linking and transparency is required and this chapter addresses this issue.

Chapter 8 – Emotional Impact: Embarrassment and Shame

Despite all the historical figures and current celebrities (Albert Einstein, Leonardo da Vinci, Muhammad Ali, Steven Spielberg, Keira Knightley, Whoopi Goldberg and Tom Cruise, to name but a few) who have been identified as dyslexic and who had or have successful lives, there still exists a 'shame' factor associated with having a specific learning difficulty. Some parents are initially too embarrassed to seek help because of the perceived stigma associated with the problem, but this only exacerbates the problem and makes it harder for the child to catch up. Initiating intervention is, for some, just too big a step to take because they must confront the academic and emotional aspects of having a specific learning difficulty. In my clinical experience, early intervention is always best, as it prevents the associated emotional and behavioural issues from taking hold. However, contrary to what I was told as an eighteen-year-old, treatment is effective at any age. Ironically, for those older students for whom profound ingrained negative emotion about their difficulty hasn't occurred, nor prevented them from accessing intervention, treatment can often be quicker and easier to administer. This is due to the fact that they have benefited from the passage of time and years of literacy exposure and experience, and in this process they will have absorbed knowledge, however disjointed that knowledge may have been. This inadvertently absorbed knowledge then simply requires attention, explanation, clarification and grounding to take hold. This chapter looks at the emotional impact of undiagnosed or diagnosed and untreated dyslexia and how to avoid any unnecessary negative effect on your child or family.

Chapter 9 – Extreme Consequences: The Dangers of Undiagnosed or Untreated Dyslexia

Having spent twelve years of my professional life working in a child and adolescent mental health service (CAMHS) dealing with many students who had emotional and behavioural problems, I am keenly aware that specific learning difficulties often have serious emotional side effects, particularly for those with a literacy problem, whether diagnosed or undiagnosed, if it has been left untreated. Many parents I interviewed expressed their concerns for their child's emotional and at times behavioural reactions to their specific learning difficulty. The aim of this chapter is to look at this issue. Specifically, it will discuss how important it is for everyone to be comfortable with differences in learning styles and to be supportive of anyone who must learn differently, so that no young person ends up distressed, depressed or in trouble as a result.

Chapter 10 – Support to Access the World of Written Words

Everyone has a right to literacy, which is profoundly important because if you can't learn to read then you can't read to learn. We live in a literate world but we also live in a fast-moving digital technology world that is changing the direction for education and teaching. We, as educators and parents, need to move with the times and understand the technology, technical skills and interests of the younger generation, who are undoubtedly technically savvy. There are now numerous ways to access materials that are available via the internet, which can assist our specific learning disabled population. This chapter explores the use of digital technology to facilitate interventions and treatments for dyslexia, and as a medium for students to navigate the 'world of written words'. It also looks at other supports available.

***

As I read my words in this opening chapter, I am struck by two thoughts. One is hope that this chapter might resonate with you, the reader, and open up a new way of viewing dyslexia for you or for anyone whom you know has had to deal with the complexity of dyslexia in their lives.

The second is my personal realisation, more vivid with every word that I write, that what often seems to be misfortune can become great fortune if we do not lose faith in ourselves. Dyslexia provided me with insights that might otherwise have been unavailable to me and deep understanding of the experience of having a specific learning difficulty; and it forced me to excavate my creativity and to discover abilities I might never have known I had.

I like to think that this book – would I ever have imagined that I might write one – will reassure anyone who is discouraged at this time by academic difference, to know that they have talent and to find it. I hope they will not lose faith in themselves, nor let anyone else lose faith in them. Intelligence is not one single thing. It is not something outside of ourselves; it is not something that is measurable in real-life terms because we are all much more than our assessment instruments can measure. Instead, I believe, that true intelligence is what we do with what we have, good and bad, advantageous and disadvantageous, burden or blessing.

If I can turn my dyslexia into a fulfilling career, spend years researching it, develop educational programmes to combat it and eventually write a book about it, then what more proof is needed that academic humiliation can be turned into self-worth. This is what made the WordsWorthLearning programme and what makes it all worthwhile for me.

What to Look For: Early Signs that Might Signal a Later Problem

Dealing with the identification and remediation or treatment of dyslexia and similar difficulties over the years, I've discovered that parents and teachers very often don't know what they don't know. They have embarked on a journey of remediation having missed early signs and signals that may have pointed to the possibility of dyslexia.

I must stress that not all signals or indicators will lead to full-blown dyslexia but they are indicative and can raise an awareness that something may need to be investigated further. Having the knowledge to recognise the early signs can prompt a parent or teacher to become more vigilant, which is imperative to ensure early identification, important prevention and, where appropriate, intervention or treatment. This could spare a child many years of failure and all the problems that go with it. Because dyslexia is so complex we can't always rely on others to recognise when there is a problem nor can we depend on our own gut instinct to recognise a problem, especially when we don't necessarily know what signs to look out for. This is particularly problematic for first-time parents and teachers or professionals who have not had the opportunity to become experienced in the diagnosis of dyslexia.

There are eight main categories to consider when trying to determine if a child has a problem, which I will explain and expand on throughout this chapter. These categories can be useful in determining if there were early signs which could indicate an emerging problem. These categories are as follows:

- Pregnancy complications and birth traumas
- Acquisition of early developmental milestones
  - Speech and language development
  - Motor and sensory development
- Family history
- Medical history
- Educational history
- Organisational skills
- Behavioural issues
- Socialisation

There is of course a plethora of useful information available in books and on the internet concerning each of the categories above. However, in my experience of interviewing thousands of parents I have been able to identify and create a checklist of possible factors that are commonly reported, which can alert you and help identify potential problems. These factors range from being exceptionally rare to commonplace. Indeed, even those without a literacy difficulty, if they were to reflect back on their own development, may have encountered some of these symptoms. Even though, at this stage there is a myriad of associated problems, I will only outline the signs that regularly appear with my clients, as they are the most accurate and offer a clear and direct path for remediation. Although there are no clear guidelines as to how many of these symptoms must co-occur to cause concern, if your child only displays one or two of these signs don't be alarmed, but if they display a number of signs across varied categories perhaps further investigation is then warranted.

Pregnancy Complications and Birth Traumas

There is still much to be discovered about the link between and impact of pregnancy problems, birth traumas and dyslexia. Although I am not an expert on the issues related to pregnancy or birth, I have noticed commonalities in the case history information provided by many parents. These include:

- Threatened miscarriage in the first or second trimester, i.e. the first three to six months of pregnancy
- Loss of a twin during pregnancy
- Trauma during pregnancy due to a serious fall or accident
- Maternal viral illness during pregnancy over and above the usual flu epidemics or similar common annual viruses
- Reported pre-eclampsia or toxaemia, which is a condition caused by very high blood pressure in the mother, resulting in fluid retention and toxins in the blood
- Excessive alcohol consumption during pregnancy, with many mothers not even being aware that they were pregnant, sometimes for up to six months
- Use of recreational drugs during pregnancy, again an issue mainly reported by mothers who weren't aware that they were pregnant at the time
- The presence of meconium (the first stool) in an infant's lungs, which the baby inhaled before delivery, often in response to foetal distress and lack of or reduced oxygen intake
- Emergency caesarean sections, often as a result of the previously mentioned conditions
- Ventouse delivery (or vacuum-assisted vaginal delivery or extraction), as a result of foetal distress

- A high forceps delivery (the use of an instrument placed at the baby's head to help guide them out of the birth canal)
- The umbilical cord being caught around the baby's neck, again leading to foetal distress
- Excessively long labour, leading to foetal distress, and in many cases the eventual need for a ventouse or emergency caesarean section delivery
- Hypoxia or anoxia, otherwise known as HIE (hypoxic-ischaemic encephalopathy), that is lack of, or the absence of, oxygen for the newborn baby, resulting in the baby being delivered a blue colour

These are the most common conditions reported. It is by no means an exhaustive list but you can use it as a trigger to consider your own personal pregnancy experience. It is important to think back and ask yourself if there was anything unusual during pregnancy or your child's birth that might have caused you some unease or concern.

Acquisition of Early Developmental Milestones

Milestones are the ages and stages at which most babies and children are expected to be able to do things, like smiling, sitting up, crawling and walking. Parents often keep a nervous eye on their baby and worry if they have not reached these milestones as quickly as other babies of that age. They are rough guidelines, e.g. walking at twelve to fifteen months, but there should not be panic if individual babies achieve these milestones in their own time. Sometimes they are so busy enjoying the experience of one new skill that another falls behind. Having said that, it is well known that there are normal developmental patterns or milestones that we can use to measure developmental progress – time periods within which we would expect a skill to appear – and if the time is exceeded greatly it can alert us to the need to monitor or assist progress in that area. There are recognised variations for these milestones that provide a tolerance for individual patterns and differences. The difficulty here is when does a developmental pattern move from normal to abnormal? When is it just too delayed, taking too long to appear, and could this significantly affect the child's ability to learn competent language and literacy skills? The early pioneering work of Mary D. Sheridan in the 1960s, after much research, clearly set out expectations for each stage of children's early development, from birth to five years of age. Her work, documented in *From Birth to Five Years: Children's Developmental Progress*,[3] has been the developmental bible for many professionals since it was first published in 1973. It has since undergone many revisions over the years. It continues to provide clear guidelines of the norms or expected times for acquiring skills, and as a result is a very useful resource for first-time parents.

With this in mind, how on earth do you determine what is normal development and what is a delay, especially when, over time, your child may catch up? In those grey areas how can you be sure that you haven't missed something that actually needs immediate attention? This is always a question for parents.

Again referring to the information provided by parents in case histories, the following early milestones are of particular significance and are a good pointer that investigation or assessment might be considered:

Speech and Language Development

- Parents report that the baby was a quiet baby, with little babbling or speech play in the early months.
- The child was slow to speak compared to their siblings or peer group.

- Parents or older siblings tend to talk for the child, demonstrating an instinctive overprotectiveness of the child. I continue to be fascinated by parents who answer for the child at the initial interview stage when the child is clearly being asked a direct question. This is the instinctive protectiveness of parents. Interestingly, on the formal language assessment testing of these children they are found, more often than not, to have an underlying language deficit.

- The child demonstrates erratic responses to sound, either not responding as expected or being overly disturbed by noises.

- The child becomes distressed or agitated in loud busy places where they seem to find it hard to sift out background noise and to focus on a particular voice or something the parent or others are saying to them. This difficulty can persist into adulthood.

- The child is overly bothered by certain noises, e.g. repetitive sounds such as whirring fans or loud bangs. This can then adversely affect their ability to concentrate on a given task in the presence of that sound.

- The child has difficulty locating a sound in their environment. They can hear it but can't detect from which direction it is coming.

- The child is presenting with indistinct or distorted speech patterns.

- The child continues to present with articulation delays or disorders beyond the age of six years, particularly with the production of /s/, /r/ or what are called digraph vowel sounds, e.g. /au, or, ar, ou/.

- They present with a limited vocabulary repertoire for their age compared to siblings or peers; this is particularly evident when children are not being read to at home and, in some cases, when they have child minders who are not fluent English speakers, which can be especially confusing for young children when they are at the stage of developing vocabulary.

- Parents or teachers often notice that a child has an immature use of grammar compared to friends or siblings of the same age.
- They experience difficulty remembering the names of common objects on command; in other words, when asked to name an item they struggle to recall a familiar word which is well within their normal vocabulary repertoire.
- They substitute words like 'thing' or 'yoke' when describing something familiar to them, e.g. 'you know that thing that you cut with' or 'can you get the yoke for cutting out of the drawer?'
- They present with a noticeably poor ability to stay on topic or keep to the subject being discussed and have difficulty in either identifying or expressing the salient point in a topic. Their thoughts and subsequent expression often wander, talking around a topic rather than being specific.
- They have difficulty retelling a story or describing events. Many parents recount situations where their child may have gone to a party or an event and, when asked about it afterwards, they were either unable or reluctant to recount any details.
- They experience difficulty learning sequences, e.g. the alphabet, days, months, seasons and times tables, and this often continues into the teenage years.
- They experience difficulty telling the time, particularly on the older analogue clock or watch faces as opposed to modern digital devices.
- They have persistent difficulty learning things by rote, e.g. poetry, rhymes, lyrics and quotations.
- They experience difficulty following verbal instructions – particularly for two and three or more element commands,

that is, if asked to do something that has more than one instruction to be completed. They would rather be shown what to do than be told what to do or to have to read instructions. I believe this is why Lego is so successful with most children of all ages and of different abilities, as the instructions are given in colourful clear diagrams and not in words.

- They have a tendency to forget or muddle instructions; it's like the information went in one ear and out the other.

- They can experience difficulty understanding humour; they just don't get the joke. Instead they can interpret what is said literally or be more concrete in their interpretation. Unfortunately, this can often lead to misunderstandings, upsets and isolation from peers. It can be confusing and upsetting not to understand why people are laughing when they themselves don't get the joke.

- They experience persistent difficulty with left and right orientation, or simply in telling right from left, and an older child might rely on memory tricks to remember directions. Some older students have ongoing difficulty following maps or giving directions.

- In general, they tend to present with poor auditory memory and auditory processing skills, but may have a good visual memory. In other words, if told to follow an instruction they may have difficulty either in remembering the detail or understanding what is expected of them. However, if shown what to do in the order required they will most likely remember the process as the image is imprinted in their visual memory.

- The student can experience difficulty processing (remembering or understanding) messages and then repeating accurately what has been said, even after rehearsals. Now, an anecdote from a few years ago: I was giving a message to a school secretary for the principal and said that I was ringing about the WordsWorthLearning programme, which was being used in the school. Strangely, she asked me to repeat my message a few times. When she insisted on repeating the message back to me I discovered the cause of the embarrassment: she had misheard or misinterpreted what I had said as the 'world's worst learning programme'. Thankfully it's not!

- Often children can seem very inattentive on auditory language-based tasks, in other words being able to listen and focus when being told something or when being given an instruction without the aid of a visual cue or hint, but these same children may spend long periods of time absorbed in visual tasks such as art activities, computer games or Lego. This shows that it is not attention that is the problem but what they have to concentrate on, or attend to, that is the source of the problem. Sadly, it can produce the idea that 'they can pay attention when they want to!' This is not what is happening, instead it is that they pay attention when they *can*.

- Older students can also continue to mispronounce more complex words, such as 'hostibal' for hospital, and sometimes use mixed metaphors, such as 'we could stand here and talk until the cows turn blue', or malapropisms, e.g. 'upsetting the apple tart'.

- Sometimes the child has already been assessed by a speech and language therapist and diagnosed with a speech and/or language deficit or impairment and has already received or is still receiving therapy.

- On the Wechsler Intelligence Scale for Children, fourth edition (WISC-IV), which is a cognitive assessment used by psychologists to measure the intellectual functioning of children from ages six to sixteen years, although their overall score on the verbal comprehension section may be within average, some of the subtest scores within this section may be erratic or down compared to the other subtests. This is often noted particularly on the vocabulary and information subtests. This will be discussed in more detail in Chapter 3.

Motor and Sensory Development

Again in this area of development there are often classic descriptions given by parents and teachers that alert us to possible problems. They are as follows:

- Baby reported to have poor muscle tone (or to have been a little floppy) as an infant.
- The child is described as having been a poor feeder or had a poor sucking reflex: they were unable to breastfeed effectively and had to be moved quickly onto a bottle.
- The child continues to be a sloppy, messy or picky eater and really dislikes certain food textures or smells.
- The child may dislike brushing their teeth.
- As a baby the child didn't crawl but bum-shuffled to get around.
- The child is reported to be either a very early walker, e.g. before ten months, or a late walker, say after eighteen months.
- The child used a walker in their first year, in which the baby sits in a wheeled frame and scoots along with their feet, thereby inhibiting crawling.
- The child was/is slow to ride a bike without stabilisers. As an older child or adult they would experience difficulty cycling from a standing upright position, or have difficulty following some of the physical cycling instructions in spinning classes at the gym.
- The child has poor balance or is clumsy in general and prone to tripping or falling.

- The child prefers sports that utilise a club, stick or racquet and can often excel in these sports, but when throwing a ball for example will more often than not miss the target.
- The child has a poor pincer grasp, that is, difficulty picking up small objects or bits of food with their fingers. At a later stage they have difficulty threading beads or tying laces.
- The child has an awkward pencil grip or cutlery grasp.
- The child has mixed dominance, in other words has not established a preference for right or left hand or foot and may use a right hand for writing but a left foot for kicking.
- The child reports that their hand tires easily. You might notice them shaking or rubbing their hand even after writing a relatively short piece or passage.
- The child demonstrates immature writing or drawing. The directionality of the letters can vary as well as the size of the text in even one sentence. Drawings can be very basic and the child may have difficulty staying within the lines when colouring in pictures.
- The child is reported to have been slow to acquire toilet training skills, and may still have accidents at night into the early teens. As a result, they are reluctant to have sleepovers or sleep anywhere other than their own bed so there is a psychological fallout too.
- The child may be poor at dressing and needs ongoing help with buttons, laces or zips. When given the choice will opt for simply designed clothing and slip-ons or Velcro-fastened shoes.
- Often children are reported to dislike labels inside clothing, which may need to be removed. An avoidance of certain fabric textures is also common. This is not being pernickety or difficult, just being sensitive to touch or textures.
- The child may have aversions to strong smells or aromas, which can trigger headaches. The occurrence of severe headaches, like migraines, is often reported with this group.

- You might see the child looking at things from odd angles, often moving the page around when reading, writing or drawing, or sometimes even moving themselves to view the page from a different angle.
- The child may have been assessed by an occupational therapist and diagnosed with dyspraxia, sensory integration difficulties, visual or auditory perceptual difficulties, or fine or gross motor difficulties.

Family History

Family history must be treated with caution. It is quite common for parents to report that dyslexia runs in their family but sometimes there are other factors which caused a reading and/or spelling difficulty that have nothing to do with genetic or biological reasons. The following, therefore, are the main factors reported that could have had an impact on the acquisition of competent literacy skills in English:

- Below average intelligence as measured formally on standardised psychological tests like the WISC-IV or Stanford–Binet Intelligence Scales
- A history of missed schooling, due to factors such as illness or frequent house moves
- Being taught using a literacy approach that didn't suit the child's learning style
- A history of fluctuating hearing loss or the presence of blocked ears after swimming under water or during a flight on an airplane
- The student attends a Gaelscoil or foreign-language school, where the teaching methods can vary greatly from mainstream English-speaking schools. This is also an educational setting in which the child is expected to learn two languages

simultaneously, which is particularly hard for a child struggling with their first language.

Just because a parent or grandparent had a literacy problem does not necessarily mean that the problem was dyslexia or there is a genetic reason down the ancestral line. In general, a more reliable indicator of a familial line is whether or not a sibling has experienced a difficulty, as in most instances they will have come from the same gene pool, will probably have attended the same pre-school or primary school and will probably have been taught using the same literacy programme being used in mainstream schools at that time.

In my clinical and personal experience, dyslexia rarely occurs in isolation. To a greater or lesser degree there will always be concomitant or associated difficulties along with the presenting literacy difficulty. If the ancestral family member also presented with some of the factors outlined earlier then there is the possibility of a family history of dyslexia. Without accurate factual information to substantiate it, I would err on the side of caution and discount a family history link. My reasons for this will be covered when I discuss the issue of labelling in Chapter 5.

Medical History

If none of the known syndromes or medical conditions outlined below that have a link to dyslexia can be identified then other reasons may account for the problems a child is experiencing. Some of the known syndromes or medical conditions are as follows:

- Foetal alcohol syndrome, a disorder that occurs when a baby is born with varied mental and physical difficulties due to the mother consuming excessive quantities of alcohol during her pregnancy

- Genetic disorders, which are disorders that occur due to genetic defects that interfere with the normal development of the body, e.g. Russell–Silver syndrome, which is a genetic growth disorder resulting in dwarfism. Although intellectual impairment or specific learning difficulties are not common with this syndrome I have had a few children with Russell–Silver syndrome and dyslexia on my caseload over the years.

- Partial complex IV mitochondrial disorder, which is a condition that depletes energy cells, particularly of the brain and muscles, causing cell damage and even cell death over the years

- Metabolic disorders, such as galactosaemia, which is a rare metabolic disorder that affects an individual's ability to metabolise the sugar galactose properly. Many children with this condition will also have general learning or specific learning difficulties.

- Attention deficit (hyperactivity) disorder, a genetic condition that affects attention span, learning and behaviour right through childhood and in many cases beyond into adulthood

- Dyspraxia, a difficulty with movement and with specific aspects of learning such as thinking, planning and carrying out sensory/motor tasks

- Autistic spectrum disorders, which are neurological disorders that affect children and adults and are identified by difficulties with social communication and interaction, and with social imagination and flexible thinking

Having read the list above, if the problem is not listed, then the problem may have arisen for other reasons, such as respiratory, ear, nose and throat problems. These are present in at least 30 per cent of the students I see, which is significant. Ear, nose and throat problems can manifest themselves through problems such as:

- Otitis media or glue ear, which may or may not lead to middle ear infections
- Tonsillitis
- Problems with adenoids
- Asthma
- Allergies like hay fever
- Rhinitis
- Glandular fever

Often students who come to me will have undergone minor surgery to remove tonsils and adenoids, or had grommets inserted. Quite a few will be on a medication to deal with these or possibly as a preventative measure. With each item on the list above fluctuating hearing can be a frequent detrimental feature, which is not always clearly identified because a full-blown infection may not have occurred. However, the impact of this unidentified infection can be significant as, for the most part, the teaching method being used in schools is predominantly an auditory one, i.e. what is called a phonic or letter–sound approach. So, if a student experiences fluctuating hearing and is being taught using an auditory or listening approach for literacy, they are partially deaf and are being taught through the sense that is not working well. As a consequence, they can miss out on fundamental literacy skills and can later present with a reading and spelling disorder similar to, but not actually, dyslexia. The difference between the two will be explained in Chapter 5.

Educational History

In the early classes in school many parents become aware that their child is showing signs of struggling with some of the literacy homework tasks, e.g. reading aloud. Discussing this can often be left until the end-of-year parent–teacher meeting. Often when the subject is raised by parents, the teacher reassures the parents that they may be overly concerned and that the child 'will grow out of it'. Of course teachers have also often met children who, for a variety of other reasons not connected with dyslexia, have caught up and it is difficult for teachers with so many pupils at different stages of development in a busy classroom to make the differential diagnosis that dyslexia requires. The problem is that while parents may be reassured, in my clinical experience children who have dyslexia don't grow out of it. They are already struggling and will continue to experience failure. I cannot stress enough how crucial it is to take action and seek advice if *any* of the following three categories applies to your child in the first few years of school:

- By the end of senior infants your child does not know the alphabet and their related speech sounds or phonemes.
- By first class your child cannot read or spell simple consonant-vowel-consonant (CVC) combination words, e.g. hat, tin, leg.
- By the end of first class your child is reluctant to independently pick up a book or engage in paired reading tasks.

Don't wait for the student to grow out of it – you need to take action as a preventative and curative measure. Don't take a chance; better to err on the side of caution than to let the problem go unnoticed.

Organisational Skills

How organised or disorganised a child is reflects important information. In my experience, students with dyslexia or related disorders tend to operate in one of two extreme ways: they are either completely chaotic and disorganised or they are super-organised and tidy. The tidy group tend to prefer routines and to plan things; as a result their lifestyle is more predictable and less stressful in the main. The chaotic group are quite the opposite, tending to be disorganised, frequently losing or forgetting things, and generally causing confusion and stress for themselves and those around them. These students inadvertently find themselves in trouble and tend to be more distressed in general.

Behavioural Issues

Parents often ask 'How can I know if my child is masking their distress?' The following list highlights the most common factors and questions you should ask yourself about your child. This topic will be covered in more detail in Chapter 8.

- Is your child avoiding situations where any literacy difficulties could be exposed, e.g. reading aloud in class?
- Are there psychosomatic complaints, e.g. headaches or sore tummies during school terms, which miraculously disappear at weekends or during holidays?
- Are they becoming either socially withdrawn or acting out, causing trouble or looking for fights within their peer group or with siblings?
- Does your child misinterpret social cues or not pick up the subtle nuances of language and get themselves into trouble or unintentionally offend or are offended by others?

- Is your child prone to bedwetting during school terms?
- Does your child need a lot of sleep or appear very fatigued during school terms?
- Does your child feel sad or angry without any obvious cause?

If some of these behaviours are evident for your child they may well be masking an underlying language or literacy difficulty, which will need to be investigated further as soon as possible.

Socialisation

This is a complex psychological subject and even in narrowing it from a literacy perspective many of the categories discussed above overlap with it in some way. By nature we are social animals and if we choose not to socialise then questions need to be asked. There are many reasons for social isolation, which can occur either by choice or for other reasons. If your child isn't integrating with their peers, or prefers to mix with either a younger age group or with adults, there must be a reason and you need to find out what that is and if it is likely to be due to any underlying emotional, educational, language or social problems. If you are unsure do seek professional help to establish the cause as in most cases a solution can be found.

***

Having read this chapter, I would hope that you have a clearer awareness and understanding of possible signs to watch out for from pregnancy onwards. The presence of these signs across the eight categories outlined should make you more aware of the possibility of a problem emerging, so that it can be assessed and treated early in order to prevent or minimise lifelong difficulties for your child.

3

TRUSTING YOUR GUT INSTINCT: WHEN TO LOOK FOR HELP

Parents frequently tell me they had a feeling something wasn't quite right. Their gut instinct told them there was something wrong but they didn't act on it; or they did act on it and their fears were allayed in the parent–teacher meeting. Deep down their concerns remained. Many parents, particularly those with younger children, report that although they felt their child wasn't progressing academically as they would have expected it was suggested by the teacher that the child would grow out of it. However, children don't always grow out of a problem and often end up requiring an assessment and intervention at a later stage if the concern is left unattended. It is never worth taking the chance. The earlier a problem is identified the sooner intervention can begin, and, in many cases, prevent a significant academic, emotional or behavioural difficulty from occurring. This is not to scaremonger but if your child is being taught at school and being read to at home and is not responding or progressing then the question should be asked *why*? You need to trust your instinct if you think something is wrong.

This is the time to go back to your child's early history, to remember the pregnancy, birth, early development, what was happening in the family, any accidents, illnesses, injuries or bereavements, everything that might have impacted on your child. For example, if a child has attended a preschool, completed junior and senior infants and by first class still has a difficulty with letter–sound correspondence or with reading or spelling of single-syllable consonant-vowel-consonant (CVC) words, e.g. bat, there is definitely a problem. This is not something the child will just grow out of. It is never too early to seek an opinion on any worry about your child. Instinct is a powerful innate sense and your instincts as a parent are invariably good. Equally, it is never too late to seek assessment and intervention; often intervention can be as much a preventative as a curative measure for literacy delays and disorders. If you take nothing else from this chapter, please heed this: act on your gut instinct. If you instinctively feel your child is struggling to develop the reading and spelling skills expected for their age and ability you will most likely be proven right. Listen to your own wisdom because nobody knows your child as well as you. You observe your child continuously, notice every detail of their development and draw comparisons between them and their siblings. Similarly, professionals often see what is not always apparent to a parent because they see so many children of the same age with similar profiles. Helping children is about listening to each other and working together for the child.

So now you are listening to your gut instinct, where do you go from here?

- Firstly, delve into your child's early history and look for all the areas that may be significant. Note these down one by one, detail by detail, because these are things that have happened and often support your concern. It's hard to dispute the facts and this will give your concern credibility, rather than you being perceived as an overly concerned parent.

- Indicate if there is a family history of speech, language or literacy difficulties, particularly in the immediate family with siblings. Document their history, i.e. where, when and what was identified; and what intervention was offered or completed for these other family members. It also helps to indicate what worked and/or didn't work for them. This may help with guiding intervention decisions and ultimately the prognosis or outcome for the child in question.
- If your child has moved school, list the schools attended, the years attended, the reason for moving and the literacy strategies and products used for your child at each of the schools.
- Indicate if your child has had any assessments carried out, e.g. medical investigations, hearing or vision assessments, or speech and language assessments. Every investigation and treatment is relevant, even those that were recommended but not availed of for whatever reason. Where appropriate make available a copy of the reports (you should always keep the original). If you don't have a report you can write to the appropriate agency or service and request one, or at the very least a summary of the findings. You are entitled to this.
- Indicate if your child has engaged in any remedial intervention, either at home, in school or with outside agencies, and the order in which they occurred. Document the name of the agency or service that provided the intervention, e.g. a home tutor, when it began, how long the intervention was given and what was covered. If you don't have this information, ask for a summary from the provider.
- Document what you do at home to help your child, e.g. do you read to your child, engage in paired reading tasks, listen to audio books, write stories, or play word search games or Scrabble?
- List your child's hobbies and talents: this is very important information when planning an intervention, e.g. is your child

artistic, are they more drawn to digital-based activities on their computer or mobile devices, are they musical?

- Describe how you perceive your child's social skills in different circumstances or environments, i.e. behaviour, attention and concentration skills, and whether they vary in different settings or with different age groups. When is your child most at ease; when most tense?

- Do you find yourself speaking or answering for your child? Do other family members do this? If so, why? Is it because instinctively you have noticed that it is hard for your child to speak for themselves?

Once you have collated this information you then need to decide what to do with it and with whom. You should begin with your child's school and ask for a parent–teacher meeting to discuss your concerns and your child's needs. Teachers, particularly those with experience, are a font of knowledge, which should be utilised. Ideally, the parent–teacher meeting should be held when the teacher has had an opportunity to get to know your child, so the first few weeks of the academic year is not an ideal time to approach a teacher, no matter how concerned you are. Prior to the meeting give the relevant information you have in a succinct and summarised form because most teachers won't have time to read copious amounts of paperwork. This should give the teacher a better understanding of your child's profile and of your own specific concerns. At the meeting try to ascertain the following from the teacher:

- Does the teacher have any concerns about your child academically, socially or behaviourally? It is important to ask about any issues, as behavioural or social problems often mask a specific learning difficulty or specific language impairment. Having worked on a multidisciplinary team in a child and adolescent mental health setting for twelve years, I never failed to be surprised at the number of children referred in with obvious emotional and behavioural issues, which were either a result of, or in association with, an underlying language or specific learning difficulty. It is sad to think that a learning difference can create an emotional problem, consequentially resulting in a young person spending so many of their early years of life being misunderstood.

- If the teacher has administered any formal standardised tests with the class, what were the outcomes and where was your child placed in relation to their peers? If not, find out when they are scheduled and exactly what assessments will be used. For some reason, many schools don't release these results until they are writing up an end-of-year school report. If a child is underperforming – no matter the degree – on any standardised school test parents should be informed as soon as it has come to light. If you don't know you can't help. Understandably, due to restricted resources schools can only provide additional help to the most severe cases, but ignoring the needs of those more mildly affected is doing those children a disservice. If the school is not in a position to provide additional assistance at least the parents can be advised on where to seek help themselves outside of the school system.

- Many schools do not administer a standardised spelling test, although in my professional view it would be most useful if they were to do so. This is because many children simply learn the spellings for the test on a Friday, but have forgotten them by the following week. This means there is no clear or accurate measurement of spelling competence and, consequently, how do you know if the child is struggling to spell to age level?

- Find out if the teacher thinks your child is underperforming and if so in what areas.

- If your child is underperforming, are they eligible for learning support and, if so, will they receive a one-to-one assessment over and above the normal class group assessment of their reading and spelling ability? If an assessment is carried out, make sure you receive a written summary of the results.
- What measures are being taken in the class to facilitate your child?
- Does the teacher feel that further professional advice should be considered, e.g. from a psychologist, speech and language therapist or occupational therapist? If so, why? If not, why not?
- If an onward referral is suggested, request that the teacher also provides a short summary of their views and concerns about your child as this will add a professional perspective and more weight to the referral.
- Finally, schedule a follow-up meeting with the teacher to keep track of progress.

When you have collated your child's relevant early developmental, medical and educational history, you will need to decide where to go next. If several professionals have been recommended, which should you see first? In my clinical experience, the three professions outside of the school system who tend to be consulted initially are psychologists, speech and language therapists, and occupational therapists. However, it should be noted that in some cases the test results from these initial assessments may indicate a further onward referral is needed, for example to:

- An audiologist to test hearing, particularly those specialising in central auditory processing disorders, which helps identify

if a child is struggling to understand what they hear, despite having normal hearing
- A behavioural optometrist, who will check if the child has a reduced ability to make sense of what they see, despite having normal vision
- A child and adolescent psychiatrist who can identify any behavioural issues or potential autistic spectrum disorders or attention deficit (hyperactivity) disorders

There is an ongoing debate surrounding the usefulness of some alternative therapies for improving literary skills. According to Elliot and Grigorenko,[4] there is a lack of convincing evidence concerning the efficacy or effectiveness of alternative interventions for improving reading and/or spelling skills. Their comments relate to:

- Physical or perceptual-motor training, e.g. Dr Martin McPhillips' Primary Movement Programme
- Visual interventions for scotopic sensitivity syndrome, e.g. Irlen lenses[5]
- Auditory interventions such as FastForWords or other similar auditory training programmes

Elliot and Grigorenko state, with multiple references to in-depth studies, that there is little evidence to show that any of these interventions are an effective means of treating complex literacy difficulties. They stress that the most effective approach to treating literacy difficulties continues to be through a systematic phonological approach that teaches the sound and letter links and rules found in the English language. From clinical experience, I would totally agree with this viewpoint.

Referral to an Educational or Clinical Psychologist

A referral to an educational or clinical psychologist is indicated when:

- There is a concern about the child's overall intellectual ability.
- There is a concern that the child is not performing at a level commensurate with or equal to their estimated intellectual ability, because they seem to be much brighter than their schoolwork is showing.
- To ascertain if the child is eligible for additional educational resources over and above the norm
- You feel there are emotional or behavioural issues with your child, or you as a parent may feel you need help managing your child. The psychologist can also identify if there are signs of autistic spectrum disorders (ASDs) or attention deficit (hyperactivity) disorders (ADHD), which may require an onward referral to a child and adolescent psychiatrist for assessment and treatment.
- They are deemed eligible for an exemption from Irish or a modern language.

If two of your child's literacy scores are at or below the 10th percentile,* then an onward referral to a psychologist is recommended as part of the process to secure a Department of Education and Skills sanctioned exemption from learning Irish in primary or Irish or a modern language in secondary school. Currently, the Department of Education and Skills requires that a student has had a full cognitive (intellectual) assessment, dated not more than two years from the application date,

---

* A percentile ranking is a comparison of a child's score within a group of 100 children of the same age; in this particular example 90 children would have performed better than a child on the 10th percentile.

which indicates they are functioning intellectually at a minimal standard score of 90 (25th percentile) and two of their attainment test scores are at or below the 10th percentile ranking for their age (i.e. tests for reading accuracy, reading comprehension, spelling or mathematics).

In primary schools these strict criteria are used for applications for formal exemption from learning the Irish language[†] and for applications to receive a formal allocation of one-to-one resource hours and learning support.

In secondary school, the situation has now changed. If a formal exemption from Irish was sanctioned in primary school this sanction will automatically be upheld for secondary school. If seeking an exemption for the first time in secondary school, then a cognitive assessment is mandatory when applying for an exemption from learning Irish or a modern language. The assessment results must clearly demonstrate that the student is within the average range of intellectual functioning and that they have two literacy scores at or below the 10th percentile ranking.

A cognitive assessment is no longer required if seeking a waiver for spelling and grammar or other accommodations for formal state examinations, e.g. the provision of a reader or the use of a word processor or other writing accommodation. However, school literacy assessments,[‡] which must be administered within twelve months of the application date, must demonstrate that the student has a standard score of 85 or less (which equates to a percentile ranking of 16 or scaled score of 7) on a Department of Education and Skills approved test. For further details please refer to the Department of Education

---

[†] See Circular 12/96 from the Department of Education and Skills.
[‡] See Department of Education and Skills Circular 0034/2015 for a comprehensive list of suitable assessments.

and Skills' *RACE Instructions for Schools 2017* document, which is available from www.examinations.ie.

The qualifying guidelines are available on the Department of Education and Skills website (www.education.ie), under 'primary circular' (Circular 12/96) for primary school children and 'post-primary circular' (Circular M10/94) for secondary school

The National Educational Psychological Service (NEPS) is linked with all schools in Ireland and provides an excellent service. However, due to limited resources, it can only cover a small number of children within the school system and must prioritise its resources and deal with the most severe cases. However, it appears that its role in secondary schools has changed since the start of 2017. Its role is now to deliver, in conjunction with the State Examinations Commission (SEC), the Reasonable Accommodations at the Certificate Examinations (RACE) information programme to schools, to provide advice and support to schools making RACE applications, and to ensure a scheme of governance and quality assurance of RACE applications is maintained. It is understood that, in the main, NEPS will no longer be administering cognitive assessments to secondary school students, as these will no longer be required for RACE applications, only for Irish exemptions. This change has only just being implemented and may be subject to modification in the future.

Should a student require a cognitive assessment and it is not being offered within the school system, parents can access a psychologist either privately or through the Dyslexia Association of Ireland (DAI). Private assessments can be expensive; although part of the cost can be claimed back from your private health insurance and/or personal tax, but do check this before confirming an appointment and make sure that you receive itemised and dated receipts. On a positive note, the waiting time for a private assessment will normally be much shorter and the sooner a problem is identified and addressed the better.

You should consult further with the psychologist before booking an educational or clinical psychology assessment:

- If the perceived gap between estimated ability and academic performance is small. In this case I would not recommend an intellectual assessment (sometimes called a psychological or cognitive assessment) because there may not be any measurable gains for the child or parent. At this stage, it would be better to get a specialist speech and language therapy assessment. The benefit here is that both language and literacy skills will be assessed and will show if a psychological assessment is required.
- If your child is under eight years of age. Unless there are other issues, I believe that a routine cognitive assessment for a younger child (eight years and under) is not always the best way forward. I have found that younger children often underperform on formal timed testing. Often when they are tested again, being older, they produce a significantly different result with a more positive profile, as they have a greater understanding of testing procedures and time constraints.

The bottom line here is, as of 2017, if you feel your child may meet the necessary criteria for a formal exemption from Irish or a modern language at school, or as a parent you need assistance for your child from an emotional or behavioural perspective, then a psychological assessment would be most useful. If your child doesn't meet the strict criteria, then knowing their IQ score is purely academic and carries no practical value other than knowing their tested ability level.

Referral to a Speech and Language Therapist

A referral to a speech and language therapist is indicated when:

- There is evidence of difficulties with speech, language, fluency (the ability to speak easily without stumbling or stuttering over words), voice (the quality or tone of voice when speaking), communication (the ability to convey a message through speech, gestures, body language, facial expressions or written words) or literacy (reading and spelling).
- There is a history of speech or language difficulties that were treated and resolved as a younger child.

  If a child is again presenting with significant literacy difficulties I have found there will often be a re-emergence of language difficulties; although, it will be a different profile to the one previously identified and resolved, as the child is older with different expectations and language demands. For example, once a seven-year-old can read the text in their book they will usually understand the content, because the language used is relatively simple and age appropriate. In contrast, an older student might be able to read accurately but doesn't understand the content because the vocabulary being used, the complexity of the sentence structures or the concepts being described may be beyond their current language level and knowledge.

- There is a scatter of scores on the Wechsler Intelligence Scale for Children IV (WISC-IV).

  The WISC-IV contains a verbal comprehension section which measures a child's ability to understand, think and learn by using language and information already known. In this section, there are five subtests: similarities, vocabulary, comprehension, information and word reasoning (the latter two are optional and are often not administered).

The WISC-IV or similar cognitive tests don't always pick up underlying language deficits, particularly if some of the subtests have been omitted. Always ask if the entire assessment or test administered to your child included all the subtests and if not ask the psychologist why they weren't included and if it would be of benefit to your child to administer them for a better language profile.

If a student's scores on the WISC-IV, as seen on the psychological report, are down on one or more of these subtests, there is a strong possibility that there is an underlying language difficulty present:

○ Similarities – which is a measure of verbal problem-solving, where a child is given two words of similar meaning and they must then describe why they are similar

○ Vocabulary – where a child names pictures and defines words read to them by the psychologist

○ Information – where a child answers general knowledge questions, drawing on long-term memory for factual information

Likewise in the working memory subsection of the WISC-IV, which measures short-term memory, i.e. the ability to take in, hold onto and reorganise lists of new information. If this is poor, there is again a strong likelihood that there is an underlying language deficit, even if the overall score is within average. I frequently find that the overall intellectual full-scale IQ (FSIQ) or general ability index (GAI) 'average' score can be influenced when there are positive scores in other subtests. For example, if a child had a score of 7 in one subtest and 13 in another subtest, then the overall average score would be 10, thus hiding the depressed score for one of the measures. This can mask an underlying language problem that may not have been picked up during the psychological assessment.

- Other areas to look out for are:
  - A difficulty with the mechanics of reading and/or spelling, e.g. understanding the three sounds /c-a-t/ when blended read or spell the word 'cat'
  - A difficulty with reading comprehension, i.e. the ability to understand what is read

  In these circumstances your child should be referred to a specialist speech and language therapist, who can provide an in-depth language and literacy assessment and remedial intervention if needed.
- If your child has a diagnosis of dyslexia, dyspraxia or ADHD there is commonly a co-morbid or coexisting presence of a language deficit[6] and the importance of an onward referral to a speech and language therapist in these cases should not be underestimated
- If your child is struggling to follow oral commands (what they are asked to do) or written instructions at home or in the classroom
- If your child experiences difficulties expressing themselves either orally (in what they say) or in written form
- If your child is experiencing difficulties with reading comprehension and is described as a reluctant reader
- If your child is experiencing difficulties with auditory memory tasks (remembering what they hear or are told) and has difficulties focusing when in noisy environments. Always keep a lookout for how your child reacts in a noisy place.

Referral to an Occupational Therapist

A referral to an occupational therapist is indicated when:

- There is a query or diagnosis of dyspraxia involving sensory integration difficulties. This includes difficulties with movement and specific aspects of learning such as thinking things through, planning, organising and carrying out motor or sensory tasks.

- There is a query or diagnosis of dysgraphia, which is a difficulty with handwriting and the ability to produce written work legibly and quickly by hand
- Your child has difficulties with self-care, e.g. dressing themselves or brushing their teeth, or with mobility
- Your child has difficulties with social function, e.g. not engaging appropriately in social situations, often appearing emotionally immature or inappropriate
- Your child has difficulties with gross or fine motor skills, such as throwing, kicking or catching a ball, hopping, skipping, jumping, riding a bike, closing buttons or tying shoe laces
- Your child's pencil grip and handwriting is poor
- If there are visual motor integration difficulties. In other words, problems integrating visual input with motor output, e.g. catching or hitting a ball. This involves seeing a ball coming towards you and then reaching out at the right time to catch it or hit it.
- If there is a difficulty with oculomotor function or eye movements. This might be a difficulty with visual tracking or 'convergence', which involves bringing the eyes closer together to follow something coming towards them at close proximity, or 'accommodation', which involves being able to switch the eye focus from long distance to short distance.
- If your child is experiencing difficulty processing sensory information, i.e. making sense of and responding to what they see, hear, smell, touch or feel around them

***

Accepting that all interviews with professionals are treated with strict client confidentiality, I would urge you to provide the fullest information possible at the time of assessment. If you withhold important information, normally from an innate sense of protection for either yourselves or your child, you should be aware that it only serves to compound the problem. Invariably the information emerges at a later stage and if it had been provided from the outset it would have facilitated a much quicker and easier intervention pathway and outcome. It is, of course, a parents' prerogative to request that certain information is not disclosed in a written report unless it is necessary for onward referral.

Dyslexia is a multi-faceted problem, requiring multidisciplinary assessments and reports that makes the whole business of assessment and treatment an exceedingly complicated process. I would always advise parents to seek appropriate clinical guidance at the earliest opportunity because there can be many stumbling blocks and obstructions along the way. You can certainly make things a bit easier for yourselves or your child by doing the following:

- Do your research.
- Collate and rationalise the information.
- Decide the starting point and order for professional assessment.
- Attend meetings supported by facts and reports. Remember, 'knowledge itself is power' (Francis Bacon).

***

This chapter covers the early indicators that should help you, as a parent or teacher, to recognise and identify if something is wrong and to act on your gut instinct as parents are usually right. You will know what information to collect and collate from your child's relevant early developmental history and their progressive educational and social progress right up to the present time. It identifies when to seek help and which professionals to seek guidance from.

It also discusses the danger of using alternative therapies to improve reading and/or spelling skills that are based on anecdotal evidence rather than research or evidence-based fact. There is no quick fix for reading and/or spelling difficulties or dyslexia, and formal literacy intervention is the best way to resolve the literacy issues that have been presented.

4

Understanding Assessments

Although I refer to the term 'dyslexia' many times throughout the book and offered an accepted definition for it in Chapter 1, there continues to be confusion regarding the term and its boundaries. The reason is that there are so many definitions out there – some concur, some conflict, some provide a broad sweep of the symptoms of dyslexia, whilst others are very specific. This lack of clarity confuses even the most experienced clinicians and teachers, never mind parents who are trying to make sense of all the terms so that they can begin to understand their own child's profile.

To make matters worse, the terminology used varies across continents. Currently, there are two terms being used worldwide:

- Specific learning disorder (from a medical perspective)
- Specific learning disability (from a psychological and educational perspective)

Dyslexia is a subcategory of both of those terms, with its own list of subskills and difficulties. Even though there is no universally agreed definition for dyslexia, the definition I think is most relevant is from page xii of the Irish *Report of the Task Force on Dyslexia* (2001), which states:

Dyslexia is manifested in a continuum of specific learning difficulties related to the acquisition of basic skills in reading, spelling and/or writing, such difficulties being unexplained in relation to an individual's other abilities and educational experiences. Dyslexia can be described at the neurological, cognitive and behavioural levels. It is typically characterised by inefficient information processing, including difficulties in phonological processing, working memory, rapid naming and automaticity of basic skills. Difficulties in organisation, sequencing and motor skills may also be present.

In addition to that formal definition, more recent definitions describe dyslexia as a subtype of a general language processing difficulty.[7] This is important because it is necessary to have a full language assessment for students who have classic dyslexia as the results obtained from the assessment are invaluable for developing an appropriate individual educational plan (IEP) for the child. The emphasis on the language processing factor in dyslexia is the most important aspect of these newer definitions because they recognise that dyslexia is not about visually seeing letters and numbers in a jumbled way – as if the problem related to visual confusion – rather it is a problem with many language-related aspects to it. Therefore, this is a complex problem that requires specialist attention.

The *Diagnostic and Statistical Manual of Mental Disorders*, fifth edition (DSM-5),[8] which is the most widely accepted nomenclature or system of names used by clinicians and researchers for the classification of mental health disorders, recommends that using a score differential between IQ and performance measurement from tests – which has been an accepted practice in the diagnosis of dyslexia for years – should no longer be used in testing for dyslexia. This means a cognitive assessment (or assessment of intelligence) to identify a child's intellectual ability will no longer be routinely required; unless there is a strong suspicion that a student is functioning well below the average range of intelligence and could potentially be classified as being in the intellectual disability range. On a more positive note, this reviewed DSM-5 classification supports a multi-disciplinary approach – with professionals from different fields working together – where joint information, including detailed client history information, as outlined in previous chapters, will now also be needed to confirm a diagnosis. Thus, there will be better and more informed treatment plans for children, which is a great advancement in understanding dyslexia.

Of course, other specific learning difficulties may be identified in a student as academic demands increase, which can have a dramatic effect on a child's academic performance. Think of it like this: if a student can't read then other school subjects, all of which require different amounts of reading, will also be affected, like Project Maths, even if the student has good general mathematical skills. This can be detected by looking at the results from psycho-educational tests such as the WISC-IV and WIAT-II UK (Wechsler Individual Achievement Test, second UK edition).

Obviously when content and context becomes more complex and technical vocabulary is being introduced then reading comprehension will almost certainly be affected. For this reason, there is a need for students to be reassessed at certain intervals so that progress can be monitored and any problems that might be developing are not missed. For instance, a problem that may have been resolved at eight years of age may re-emerge with different patterns at a later stage in the child's development, exposing the divergent and changing profile of their specific learning difficulty over time, or, in other words, underlying problems show themselves in different ways at different times throughout a child's primary, secondary and third-level education.

As the definition of dyslexia is confused by diagnostic criteria, it stands to reason that there is no present consensus on the actual number of people with dyslexia because the numbers change depending on which definition is taken. There are different numbers published globally by interested parties, which range from 5 per cent of the world's population to a staggering 20 per cent. Nowadays, it is generally accepted that up to one-third of the school-age population are underperforming on reading and spelling tasks; however in reality only a much smaller percentage are presenting with classic dyslexia. The remainder (who are not dyslexic) present with reading/spelling delays or disorders resulting from situations that are neither neurological nor genetic/biological in origin and are more likely to be a consequence of what I believe are the three primary causes:

- They have an overall lower IQ but are not in the intellectual disability range.
- The teaching method used in their school doesn't suit their learning style.
- They suffered from fluctuating hearing loss during some key stages of literacy teaching.

Although all three of the above fit under the 'specific learning disability' label, the term 'dyslexia' is not synonymous with or exactly the same as a reading and/or spelling disorder, disability or delay. Dyslexia has a unique and defined set of factors or characteristics which sets it apart from other labels. This is a fundamental and exceptionally important point, which I will expand on and explain in greater detail in Chapter 5.

However, for ease of explanation at this juncture the fundamental points are that the presence of a specific learning difficulty can only be diagnosed and categorised following a battery of tests, usually administered by a multidisciplinary group of professionals, i.e. teachers, psychologists, speech and language therapists and occupational therapists. The results from these tests are essential in order to take full consideration of a child's individual profile and identify the most appropriate intervention or help that specific child needs. Although this multidisciplinary approach does appear to be 'taking a sledgehammer to crack a walnut', especially when not all interventions are required, the benefits of doing a full multidisciplinary profile are that results will provide a detailed picture of the child early on, allowing for a more immediate, focused and accurate intervention to resolve the literacy difficulty. Put simply, the more information we have from different perspectives on the child's development, the more specific and tailor-made will be the help the individual child gets. The right help for the right problem at the right time is the key.

Unfortunately, and understandably, the overall cost of the assessments can be a problem for parents. Thus, some of the recommended assessments may be delayed in the hope that time will solve the problem; although in reality this normally results in the child falling further behind in school. There are other reasons why assessments are delayed, apart from the cost, for example the reluctance of the child to be assessed, because sometimes parents and child can feel overwhelmed by the whole situation and do not feel up to all that assessment and diagnosis require. While fully understanding this dilemma, it cannot be said too often that there are genuine dangers in delaying assessment. It concerns me how often, almost as a norm, students are attending my service as late as one to two years after the initial recommendation was made, be it from the school, psychologist or occupational therapist. The postponement only worsens the problem for the child. The lapsed time increases the gap where the child is falling behind the peer group and not achieving to his or her potential. Falling behind causes emotional distress, makes everything at school harder and affects the child's self-esteem. As stated previously, if a problem is flagged at all then act on it immediately as the child will not grow out of it. Literacy problems and the emotional consequences will only become more severe as time passes without the correct intervention.

The order of scheduling of appointments for the multidisciplinary assessments is important. I can honestly say that I am aware of a major improvement with the communication and joint work between the key multidisciplinary professionals that I work with: speech and language therapists, psychologists, teachers and occupational therapists. The benefits from this approach are significant because it joins the dots between the different professions, accelerating remediation for the child instead of it being stretched out over long periods of time. Thus, problems are being identified and worked on sooner and more comprehensively now than they were before, lessening the long-term negative impact on the child.

Recently I was exchanging emails with a most concerned mother who described herself as being 'mithered' over what to do for her teenage son. Although she had been given lots of advice from different sources she found most of it conflicting and confusing. With limited financial resources she wanted to do the best for her child and she made it quite clear that for every investment made there needed to be a positive gain as something had to be sacrificed in the family budget to fund it.

This set me thinking in general about how I could simplify and explain best the complexity of the assessment process to people because so many people are confused by what they are told and frustrated by conflicting advice. I then set about designing a chart to show the options that should be considered and the procedure to identify the correct assessments that could be carried out and how they all interlink. This will hopefully make things much clearer for a concerned parent, caregiver or professional and put them on the right path. Parents should also remember that the best place to start if they have any worries or questions is to arrange a parent–teacher meeting, where they can talk about their concerns and hear what the teacher thinks. At the meeting they should try to identify which professional to begin with, i.e. the psychologist, speech and language therapist or occupational therapist. The flow chart opposite should help with that process.

Understanding the assessment process: The box in the far left of the diagram identifies the professional to be involved first, the next box identifies the factors to be considered when choosing that path, the third box informs you what assessment(s) will be required with the possible recommendations for follow-up assessment(s), and the final box gives some reasons why that particular assessment is important.

At the end of each academic year schools are obliged to give parents a report containing the standardised test results for their children. These tests are a measure of a child's achievement compared to other children in all schools at the same class level or age level. Most parents don't fully understand what a standard score, standard deviation, STen score or percentile rank means and the implications that these scores might have for their child in terms of qualifying for extra resources or accommodations in school. So, before going any further, we need to have a look at the importance of the scores and what they are telling us about the child. Let's start with the basic terms being used:

1. *Standard score*: This is another way to show where a child is placed in comparison to others of the same age. A standard

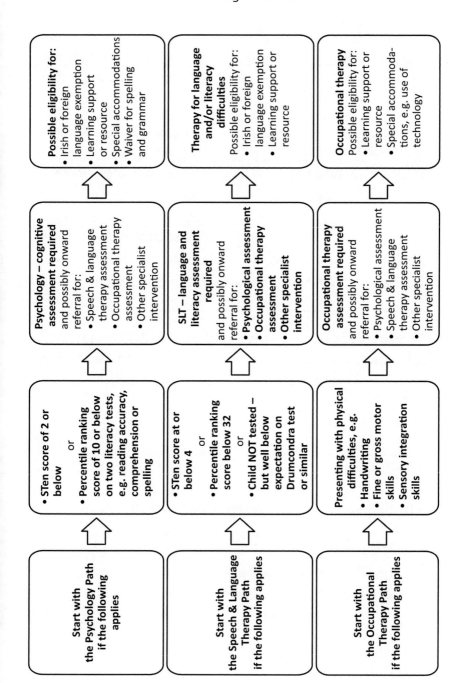

Start with the Psychology Path if the following applies

- STen score of 2 or below

  or

- Percentile ranking score of 10 or below on two literacy tests, e.g. reading accuracy, comprehension or spelling

Psychology – cognitive assessment required and possibly onward referral for:

- Speech & language therapy assessment
- Occupational therapy assessment
- Other specialist intervention

Possible eligibility for:

- Irish or foreign language exemption
- Learning support or resource
- Special accommodations
- Waiver for spelling and grammar

Start with the Speech & Language Therapy Path if the following applies

- STen score at or below 4

  or

- Percentile ranking score below 32

  or

- Child NOT tested – but well below expectation on Drumcondra test or similar

SLT – language and literacy assessment required and possibly onward referral for:

- **Psychological assessment**
- **Occupational therapy assessment**
- **Other specialist intervention**

Therapy for language and/or literacy difficulties

Possible eligibility for:

- Irish or foreign language exemption
- Learning support or resource

Start with the Occupational Therapy Path if the following applies

Presenting with physical difficulties, e.g.

- Handwriting
- Fine or gross motor skills
- Sensory integration skills

Occupational therapy assessment required and possibly onward referral for:

- Psychological assessment
- Speech & language therapy assessment
- Other specialist intervention

Occupational therapy

Possible eligibility for:

- Learning support or resource
- Special accommodations, e.g. use of technology

score of 90 is the start of the average range, which is equal to a 25th percentile ranking. A standard score of 110 is the upper end of the average range and is equal to a percentile rank of 75. The following table shows each of the ranges:

Standard Score (SS)	Category	Compared to Age Group
115 or above	Well above average	Top one-sixth of students
108–114	High average	One-sixth of students
93–107	Average	Middle two-sixths or one-third of students
85–92	Low average	One-sixth of students
84 or below	Well below average	Bottom one-sixth of students

2. *Standard deviation*: This is a statistical method for calculating where the child is placed in the average band, i.e. ranging from well below average to well above average. The following table shows each of the ranges:

Standard Deviation (SD)	Category	Compared to Age Group
+1.5 SD and above	Well above average	Top one-sixth of students
+1 to + 1.5 SD	High average	One-sixth of students
Within + or - 1 SD	Average	Middle two-sixths or one-third of students
-1 to -1.5 SD below	Low average	One-sixth of students
-2 SD and below	Well below average	Bottom one-sixth of students

3. *STen score*: simply means a Score out of Ten, which is another way of comparing your child's performance against other

children at the same age level. The following table explains each of the ranges and their equivalent percentile ranking scores: If your child's STen score is 5 or 6, you will know that his/her performance on the test is average. About one-third of children in Ireland have STen scores in this band. You can see from the table that there are also STen scores above and below the average.

STen Score	Percentile Rank	Category	Compared to Age Group
8–10	85th–100th	Well above average	Top one-sixth of students
7	67th–84th	High average	One-sixth of students
5–6	33rd–66th	Average	Middle two-sixths or one-third of students
4	16th–32nd	Low average	One-sixth of students
1–3	1st–15th	Well below average	Bottom one-sixth of students

4. *Percentile ranking (PR)*: Comparing a group of 100 students of the same age, a PR score from a standard assessment indicates where each student has been placed within that group. On most standardised tests the average scores range from the 25th to the 75th percentile rankings. So, if your child scores in the 25th percentile (the bottom end of average) there would be 75 in the group above with a better score and 24 in the group below with a lesser score. We will explore this in more detail later in this chapter.

Over the years, I have been developing and refining the graph shown on page 62. I use it after an assessment to explain to the parents where their child is performing and to also let them know if they might be eligible for learning support or other

AGE EQUIVALENT – PERCENTILE RANKING and STen SCORES for READING and SPELLING

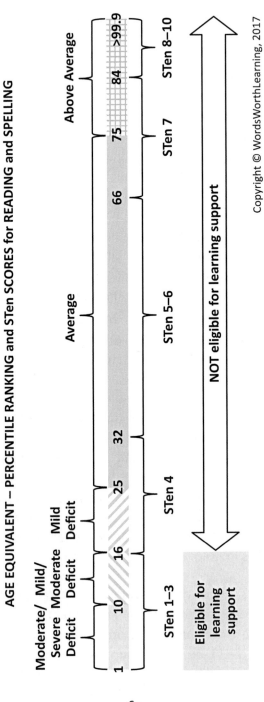

accommodations. Interestingly, many parents comment that it is the first time they have understood the results. This chart can also be applied for assessments administered by other professionals.

So how does this chart work? Firstly, if you child has had a psychological/cognitive assessment done they will have been given either a full-scale IQ (FSIQ) score or a global ability index (GAI) score and corresponding percentile ranking. I suggest you mark this percentile ranking score on the chart; the number will be somewhere between 1 and >99.9. Keep in mind that the results from tests administered are only indicators of performance on the day and scores can fluctuate depending on age, mood, state of health and even how comfortable your child felt at the time of testing.

Results are not cast in stone, as a case in point demonstrates: many years ago, I assessed a young girl who was diagnosed as being on the autistic spectrum. As a pre-schooler she had initially been tested as functioning low in the moderate range of intellectual disability; hence, from her test results it looked as though she was of low intelligence. Because of severe language and communication difficulties she was unable to perform as expected on standardised tests at that young age. She then went on to receive extensive intervention from a number of services. I first met her when she was a teenager and she presented with diagnosed Asperger's syndrome, a specific language impairment, dyslexia and dyspraxia. Following the previous intensive intervention she had received and the amazing endless support from her mother, I could see her profile had changed significantly, and although she could demonstrate her intellectual potential she was still struggling to achieve her academic potential. At that stage, she did the WordsWorthLearning programme with me and made significant gains in reading, equalling her intellectual ability; although her spelling remained a problem, albeit less severe. Additionally, from the recommendations in her occupational therapy assessment she was able to avail of assistive technology to support her written work, which alleviated the spelling problem, so it didn't hold her back. Over the years her profile and diagnosis had changed dramatically, which was clearly evident after a cognitive reassessment that was carried out in her fifth year at secondary school, when she was found to be functioning in the superior range of intellectual ability. She is now a qualified and employed paramedical professional, with a good honours degree from Trinity College Dublin. The lesson to be learned from this extreme case is that a child's profile and diagnosis can change dramatically over time, and with the correct intervention the results can be life-changing. This particular girl was very fortunate to have had access to all the available remedial services, which I believe was largely due to her mother's tenacity. Had this not been the case I wonder where she would be now.

Returning to the chart, it was designed to help identify if a child would be eligible for accommodations, i.e. special arrangements made for students with permanent or long-term conditions, such as visual and/or hearing difficulties and specific learning difficulties. Examples of accommodations include a waiver for spelling and grammar, in exceptional cases extra time in exams, or the provision of a reader or scribe. These accommodations can be used to facilitate students whilst taking lessons, lectures, studies and state examinations.

The chart is also used to indicate if there might be a requirement for a cognitive assessment, i.e. would there be any benefit other than knowing the IQ score. For a score at or below the 10th percentile the child is presenting with a moderate to severe difficulty in one or more of the following areas: language skills, reading accuracy, reading comprehension, speed of reading, spelling or mathematics. To be eligible for language exemptions this score must be evident in two or more of the literacy attainment assessment tests and, from a language perspective, a student must also be functioning two standard deviations below the norm, i.e. the equivalent of a STen score of 1–2 or a percentile ranking score of 1–10. If this is the case, a cognitive assessment will be required when applying to the Department of Education and Skills for a language exemption.

A score between the 11th and 16th percentiles means the child is presenting with mild to moderate difficulty. Up until January 2017 they were not eligible for any additional resource hours in school; although in some schools it was discretionary and this usually depended on the needs and resources that were available within the school. Since January 2017, if a child scores at or below the 16th percentile or achieves a standard score of 85 or less, they are now eligible for learning support in school. This change has been sanctioned for 2017 only and may change again in coming years.

Scores between the 17th and 25th percentiles indicate a mild difficulty and students within this range are not eligible for additional resources hours in school.

The average band ranges between the 25th and the 75th percentile rankings and of course a child within this range would not be eligible for extra help. Herein lies a problem: if a child has tested with an IQ at the 60th percentile and their literacy test scores are at the 30th percentile there is a very big gap between their intellectual potential and their actual performance. To all intents and purposes, they are regarded as being in the average range and performing normally. In my opinion, this is a child who is underperforming and unlikely to reach their academic potential. I have seen many students with profiles like this, where their intellect suggests that they have the ability to deal with more advanced material, but their actual reading ability is holding them back. I have also, over the years, come across a number of exceptionally bright students in the gifted range whose literacy scores are at the average range. They are unfortunately caught in a system that misses the issue because if their reading skills were improved they would be able to perform to their academic potential.

Sometimes parents begin to panic when their child has been retested in school on tests such as the MICRA-T (Mary Immaculate Reading Attainment Test) or the Drumcondra reading tests and their child's STen scores are either the same or below those obtained the previous academic year. To put it in context, if a child obtains a STen score of 5 in fourth class and again scores a 5 in fifth class, a parent can assume that no progress has been made. This is an incorrect assumption because the test material would be age appropriate and would be more difficult than the previous year, so the student has made steady progress and has improved by the margin expected within the one-year span; so, in other words, their academic ability has remained consistent. On the other hand, using the same example, if the score dropped from a STen of 5 to a 4 this indicates that no observable progress has been made, but it is important to recognise that the child hasn't lost any skills; they just haven't gained any ground in the year.

In summary, my advice to parents would be:

- Ask the school for the STen score and the percentile ranking score, so you can find out exactly where your child is on the percentile/STen graph.
- If you have your child's IQ score, compare this with their tested literacy ability score. They should be in or around the same score and if this is not the case you must question why and follow it up with the school.
- If the scores are below the 10th percentile ranking on two of the literacy-related tests, speak with the school principal

and learning support teacher and find out what supports and exemptions your child may be eligible to receive.

- Keep in mind that timing is important when making an application for resources; move quickly because it is possible that your child could move out of this range and the opportunity could be missed with a late application, which may then not be approved.

- If your child's scores are at or below the 10th percentile on two literacy-related tasks, seek a cognitive assessment (if you don't already have one) either through the school or privately. This is required for a formal exemption from learning Irish.

- Unfortunately, many schools are burdened with under-resourced learning support services and are unable to provide a service for those students whose needs are not sufficiently severe. You should be aware that if your child has a score between the 17th and 32nd percentile ranking and/or a STen score of 4 or less, and you are concerned that they have a reading and/or spelling difficulty that is holding them back, you should seek a referral for a detailed language and literacy assessment, ideally from a speech and language therapist who specialises in literacy delays and disorders. Many of my clients are from this cohort and after remediation they overcome their difficulties and go on to achieve better academic outcomes.

***

This chapter has shed some light on the complex area of multidisciplinary assessments. It has looked at which professional services should be involved and when is the most opportune time to seek help.

The chapter has provided some guidelines for understanding and selecting appropriate professional assessments and explained some of the complexities surrounding assessment scores and how they impact on eligibility for services.

The chapter also emphasises and explains the importance of understanding the percentile ranking and STen score results and what it means for the academic future of your child. In doing so it suggests that the assessment and diagnosis process is merely a snapshot that reflects the measurement and evaluation of any symptoms or behaviours at a specific point in time. Some of these may never alter but others can change dramatically, especially with a coordinated, multidisciplinary approach that also includes a strong and determined parental contribution.

5

WHEN IS DYSLEXIA NOT DYSLEXIA

The term 'dyslexia' is used excessively and often incorrectly. Unfortunately, it has become a convenient and socially acceptable catch-all label for every kind of difficulty associated with reading and writing without proper differentiation between classic dyslexia and a reading and/or spelling delay or disorder. Liberally applying the label dyslexia is misleading and it can also be damaging for someone to be labelled as dyslexic when in fact they have a lesser condition that is capable of being fully remediated. Of course the dyslexic label may appear to fit a profile fairly well and is therefore convenient but the question is this: is near enough good enough and does it really matter? The answer to that question is that it does matter because labels have a deeper meaning and consequence.

The significance of labels can be shown by an incident that occurred recently involving an elderly friend of mine who was admitted to hospital at short notice for specialist tests. This required being an in-patient for several days, and because my friend had been advised to increase her fluid intake she hurriedly packed bottles of soft drinks for her bedside locker: a bottle of fizzy elderflower water and a bottle of Cidona. After settling in at the hospital she was horrified to discover, as were her accompanying family members, that the bottle of Cidona displayed on the bedside locker was actually a bottle of strong cider. She had misread the label and bought it by mistake. Given the circumstances and the message it might convey, it was hidden quickly. The point is that a label demonstrates or describes the content and ultimately the impact or consequences resulting from it. In a similar way, to be labelled as dyslexic is only of benefit if it is accurate and fitting. Other reading and/or spelling disorders can have similar characteristics to dyslexia but they are not the same as dyslexia because, unlike dyslexia, they can be completely remediated or resolved. From a clinical perspective, if the label isn't accurate then it should not be used; if it is accurate then it should be used for the benefit of the person with the condition. A label should be a way of explaining and validating the genuine struggle a person has with an identifiable condition. It should be a positive, practical, accurate and supportive description.

Parents who attend my practice quite often use the term 'dyslexic' for their child because the child's level of reading and/or spelling is not as high as they think it should be for their age and estimated or known ability. It cannot be said often enough that poor reading and/or spelling skills does *not* necessarily mean the child is dyslexic and it is important that children are not mislabelled. From experience, at this stage of my life I embrace my label of dyslexia in a very positive way because I see it as a key part of my identity. To be honest, this is only after years of struggling and feeling both shame and embarrassment about being dyslexic with literacy difficulties. I now accept the strengths it brings me, in tandem with the obvious ongoing deficits, which I now fondly regard as quirks of my personality.

Even today there is a lot of general ignorance and confusion surrounding dyslexia, but this is changing as governments worldwide are introducing educational policies that will hopefully level the playing field for all students with such difficulties.

At last tags such as 'stupid', 'slow' or 'backward' are disappearing as it is now recognised that many dyslexic people are intellectually bright with high IQs. These much-needed changes in attitude will take time and the fact still remains that when someone is labelled as dyslexic they are treated as if they are less intellectually able. The message should be that they are just as intelligent as their classmates; they just need a different approach to learning and, in some cases, require special accommodations to help them in examinations. I regret to say that, even today, some people (including professionals) who should know better make incorrect assumptions about the academic capacity and potential of a person once they know they are dyslexic. This is so wrong. When someone with dyslexia is taught by focusing on their learning strengths they can excel, often beyond that of their mainstream peers.

The experience of working with thousands of students with literacy difficulties and their parents has given me an acute awareness of the confusion that abounds. I have developed a three-tier classification diagram that explains the term 'specific learning difficulty', showing the multi-layered aspects of the

THREE-TIER CLASSIFICATION MODEL ©			
Specific Learning Difficulty (SLD)			
Developmental Dyslexia *or* Reading/Spelling Disorder			
DECODING/ ENCODING DISORDER	ORAL LANGUAGE PROCESSING DISORDER	WRITTEN LANGUAGE PROCESSING DISORDER	MIXED SYMPTOMS
difficulty with knowing how to read and spell	difficulty with understanding or using language	difficulty understanding what is read	presenting with aspects from all three

condition and defining what it is. It does provide some clarity and has helped parents to understand where their child is placed in the scheme of things.

If a student is diagnosed with developmental dyslexia or a more general reading/spelling disorder both difficulties would be classified under the umbrella of a specific learning difficulty. However, a student with a reading and/or spelling disorder would experience difficulties primarily with decoding and/or encoding skills, while the dyslexic student would be in the 'mixed symptoms' group, thus experiencing difficulties, to varying degrees, across all three parameters.

The following case studies give an example of the diagnostic complexity and how to apply test results using this model. In order to protect clients' confidentiality, identifying details for the clients involved have been omitted and their names have been changed.

Katie's Story

Katie is a nine-year-old girl, the eldest of three children. Following a difficult pregnancy for her mother, she was delivered through an emergency caesarean section because both mother and baby were in distress. Katie's early developmental milestones were normal except for the fact that she didn't crawl but bum-shuffled until she was eighteen months old. Her language development was also delayed, but she was never referred for speech and language assessment prior to attending my service, at nine years of age. Although her gross coordination skills were thought to be normal, her handwriting was poor and she was left-handed. A cognitive assessment (or assessment of her intelligence) was carried out by a NEPS educational psychologist and, because there was a wide scatter of scores on her WISC-IV profile, only her

GAI score was given, which was in the average range of ability. Katie's working auditory memory (remembering what she had heard) was particularly poor; although her visual skills were very strong. Katie is very artistic. All of her reading, spelling and mathematical test scores were under the 10th percentile for her age, which means that in a group of 100 children of similar age she would be performing in the bottom 10 of that group. Katie was diagnosed with 'specific learning difficulty/ dyslexia' and an exemption from studying Irish was recommended and approved by the Department of Education and Skills. At this point a speech and language assessment had still not been recommended. Katie had also been seen by a child and adolescent psychiatrist and was diagnosed with an attention deficit disorder (ADD). She had been attending learning support since senior infants and continues to receive it. Katie's mother reported that, from year to year, no observable improvements had been noted and the scores on her last Drumcondra reading and spelling test (which are tests given in primary school) were in the low range. That score was prior to attending my service.

Katie was referred to me only after her family had heard about my online WordsWorthLearning programme from other parents in her school. This was nearly two years after the initial psychological assessment. From my speech and language assessment she was found to have the following:

- A severe receptive language (comprehension) impairment, i.e. difficulty understanding what is said to her
- A severe auditory memory difficulty, i.e. difficulty remembering what she heard
- Very poor vocabulary knowledge or poor understanding of words
- Her reading continued to be in the severely disordered range.

- Her reading comprehension, or understanding what she read, was in the mild to moderate disorder range.
- Her spelling continued to be in the severely disordered range.
- Her written composition was illegible.

Katie needed specific help. At the time of writing Katie is midway through therapy and is progressing well, and academic improvements have been noted both at home and in school.

Considering Katie is in the average range of intelligence but with reading and spelling skills way below expectation, and that she has been diagnosed with a specific learning difficulty, the question is: does she have developmental dyslexia or a reading/spelling disorder? To be very clear, it should be one or other, it *cannot* be both and it is very important to know which one. Although the therapy may be similar, the length of therapy and the outcomes will vary according to the severity of the problem.

What we know:

- She had a traumatic birth and her developmental history shows significant difficulties.
- From standardised literacy tests we know she has a decoding/encoding disorder, in other words she has difficulty knowing how to read and spell.
- From language assessment tests, we know she has a severe comprehension disorder or difficulty understanding what is said to her. She also has poor memory and poor vocabulary knowledge.
- From literacy tests, we also know that she has difficulty understanding what she reads.

Putting all this information together, and using the three-tier classification model above, we can determine that Katie has dyslexia because she has difficulties across all three sections, showing a mixture symptom profile. Katie is presenting with a specific learning difficulty which is dyslexic in nature.

John's Story

John is a bright eleven-year-old boy, the second of four children. His mother reported that her pregnancy with John was normal and she had a standard delivery. All of John's developmental milestones were reported to be normal to advanced. John's medical history was normal; he was neither on medication nor was he under the care of any medical specialist. His hearing and vision were both tested and found to be normal. There was no family history of dyslexia or of language impairments in the immediate or extended family. John was described as being very well coordinated and good at sports. He is both artistic and musical. John attends a Gaelscoil and is fluent in Irish for his age. In 2012 John underwent a psychological/cognitive assessment and was found to be functioning in the high average range of intellectual ability, with normal to high scores across the four parameters or sections on the WISC-IV intelligence test. On literacy attainment tests his scores were just above the 10th percentile, showing that he had difficulties with knowing how to read and spell. His reading comprehension score was under the 10th percentile and he also struggled with the written aspects of both Irish and English. John was diagnosed with a 'specific learning difficulty/dyslexia' by the educational psychologist and learning support was recommended and approved.

Before he was referred to my service, John had the following interventions:

- He attended Dyslexia Association of Ireland (DAI) workshops every Monday night for two hours, for over a year.

- He attended learning support twice a week, in a small group, using the Toe-by-Toe and SNIP literacy programmes. He was also using the look-cover-write-check strategy for spelling, which is a spelling technique commonly used in most primary schools in Ireland.
- He also had a home tutor who came to his house once a week for an hour.

John was referred to my service, again, only after the family had heard about my online WordsWorthLearning programme from other parents in his school. John was seen for initial assessment at the end of 2012. On assessment John was found to have the following:

- Above average language skills, which were in keeping with his high level of intellectual ability
- Excellent auditory memory skills
- Advanced vocabulary knowledge
- His reading accuracy was in the mildly disordered range.
- He presented with an associated mild reading comprehension delay, in other words if he could only read the text accurately he would understand the content.
- His spelling was in the mild to moderate disordered range.
- Concerning written expression, John wrote an informative passage with a clear sequence of thought. Interestingly, it had multiple spelling errors, e.g. 'redy' for 'ready', 'afftur' for 'after', 'finisht' for 'finished'. The words were phonetically correct but the spelling was wrong.
- John's handwriting was good.

Following my language and literacy assessment, it was agreed that all other interventions should be put on hold because I didn't want him to become any more confused using various intervention methods. John attended for twelve therapy sessions and used the online WordsWorthLearning programme at home. The sessions were spread between January and October 2013 with a three-month summer break in the middle. A year later, at his parents' request, John attended my service for an additional three revision sessions to reinforce the more advanced concepts of the programme. Some weeks after completing the programme, John was then seen for a literacy reassessment in December 2014. The results after reassessment were as follows:

- John's reading accuracy skills had moved from the 30th percentile to the 89th percentile; he was now performing over two years ahead of his actual age whereas before he had been thirteen months behind.
- His reading comprehension moved from the 30th percentile to the 70th percentile; he was now performing just under two years ahead of his actual age whereas before therapy he was eleven months behind.
- His spelling skills had moved from being nearly three years behind his actual age to being within average, although still a year and a half behind.
- Following an intensive revision of the spelling rules John's spelling skills are due to be reassessed again in the near future.

Considering John is in the high average range of IQ and his reading and spelling skills were well below expectation for his tested intelligence and he has been diagnosed with a specific learning difficulty, the question is: does John have developmental dyslexia or a reading/spelling disorder?

What we know:

- John's early history was totally normal.
- From testing we know he had a decoding/encoding disorder (a difficulty with knowing how to read and spell).
- From language testing we know he has advanced language skills, so there was no difficulty in this area.
- From literacy testing we also know that he does not have difficulty understanding what he reads.

You can be fairly sure that if the reading comprehension scores are at or above a child's ability to read it demonstrates that if the child could read the passage without difficulty they would not have a problem understanding it. It was also interesting to note that once John's reading accuracy improved his reading comprehension skills also improved. As John only had difficulty in the decoding (reading) and encoding (spelling) sections it is my opinion that he is *not* dyslexic, even though he was initially referred with a diagnosis of dyslexia due to his reading and spelling difficulties. John's difficulties were compounded by the fact that he attended a Gaelscoil where the method used to teach English literacy did not suit his particular learning style. Also, English literacy skills are taught at a later stage in the curriculum of Gaelscoileanna than they would be in an English-speaking primary school. I believe these factors to be the origin of John's initial difficulty.

***

When teaching something new to a bright student like John, he understands and retains ideas and concepts quickly and immediately puts them into practice. But do keep in mind that spelling is a far more complex task than reading and so it normally takes longer to improve spelling skills. This is simply because when you are reading a word it is there in front of you to decode, but when you are trying to spell a word you have to think about the many parts involved such as sounds, letters, rules, syllables, prefixes and suffixes. I'm sure that John will not need further help from my programme after his review assessment and I would be very surprised if he needs to come back to me for help in the future.

In contrast, I know that Katie will need to be monitored over time to ensure that associated difficulties don't re-emerge and if they do they should be dealt with immediately. Keeping a keen eye on her progress will prevent other problems from developing as she gets older and academic demands increase.

So a conundrum: when a student has been diagnosed with dyslexia, which by definition is a life-long condition, and after treatment the student is functioning above their age level and no longer has a problem – as is the case with John and many others I have worked with – are they or were they ever dyslexic? I believe not.

Katie has classic dyslexia and although I anticipate significant improvements over time and think she will achieve academically, her dyslexia will be with her for life and this will be obvious at times during her development. It is clear that wise subject choices in school will be very important for her. She is a practical child and good at Art; subjects like Geography, Home Economics, Biology and Computer Studies will suit her learning style as they are factual and visual. Language-based subjects will pose significant difficulties for her as she continues with her struggle. However, she has an exemption from Irish and will also get exemptions in the future for modern languages if needed. With a diagnosis of dyslexia students can avail of formal exemptions and accommodations for state examinations and also for third-level colleges if they are scoring below the 10th percentile on two literacy tasks, so keep this in mind and always retain a copy of any assessment reports you ever receive on your child as these will be required at a later stage as proof of how long-standing the difficulties have been.

I believe John was mislabelled as dyslexic but he continues to use the label 'dyslexic' even though there is no evidence of him having that difficulty. Bizarrely, his school still regards him as being dyslexic although he is now top of his class in all subjects and does not warrant or need any extra help in school. John's parents, very wisely, do not see him as being dyslexic and do not use that label. They have altered their academic expectations for him and now expect him to achieve to his academic potential.

Considering all of the above, my advice is this: if the hat fits wear it; if it doesn't hang it up.

***

This chapter describes the confusion that abounds from the overuse of the term 'dyslexia'. It provides a three-tier classification diagram that explains the term 'specific learning difficulty', showing the multi-layered aspects of the condition and what they mean. It helps to identify the type of reading and spelling delay or disorder a person may have, which is explained in detail using two genuine case studies. Correct diagnosis is extremely important for the student and for managing academic expectations and planning a person's academic path through the education system.

6

CHOOSING THE RIGHT HELP

We live in a world where manufacturers make promises about their products. Let us consider a marketplace that is bombarded with educational products all claiming to be the 'panacea' for dyslexia or some other reading or spelling difficulty. There are so many products and materials on the market today that school policymakers, teachers and parents alike (not to mention the children themselves) are totally confused by it all. On top of that, considering all the different remedial approaches on offer, choosing the correct one has become mind-boggling to say the least. The good news is that there are some proven and researched programmes available that provide compensatory strategies to help with listening, visual and motor skills that may improve a student's ability to:

- Concentrate and listen to auditory information – the ability to focus on and understand language that you hear
- Strengthen eye tracking and movement – the ability of the eye muscles to allow a person to visually focus on objects that are near or far or are moving from side to side
- Improve fine and gross motor skills – the skills required to be able to do fine movements like picking up a crumb with your

thumb and index finger or larger movements like hopping, skipping and jumping

It is important to keep in mind that, despite claims to the contrary, none of these programmes will 'cure' dyslexia or similar reading/spelling disorders. They are physical interventions, which on their own will not give students the required strategies to be able to read and spell competently, but many can be useful in helping to alleviate some of the associated problems.

So, the big question is where do you begin? I am constantly dealing with a variety of literacy interventions and approaches that are being used in schools or private services that quite simply do not work and never have worked. The Irish National Council for Curriculum and Assessment (NCCA) provides statistics which show that more than 30 per cent of students attending primary and secondary school today have at least some degree of difficulty with reading and spelling. The majority of the interventions that are used with this group do not justify the time, money and effort expended on them. What is consistent though is the extent to which many of the students taking these school remedial programmes have been failing and how many switch off and opt out of the educational system because it is not working for them. They suffer from poor self-esteem. Sometimes parents tell me that if the school remedial programme hadn't worked first time around for their child, the same remedial programme was used again, only at a slower pace.

The question here is why? If it didn't work the first time around, why do it again? If whatever had been used didn't work then you as a parent need to take action, talk to the teacher and look for a programme that *does* suit your child's individual profile and learning style. As Albert Einstein once said, 'insanity is doing the same thing over and over again and expecting different results', which is a thought worth keeping in mind. Don't let your child be taken down a route that doesn't work for a second or even a third time. If it doesn't fit, forcing it will not change that.

There are many myths and misunderstandings about dyslexia. For example, many people think that we dyslexics see letters and words backwards. In my experience, reversing letters when either reading or writing isn't necessarily a sign of dyslexia because young children who don't have dyslexia sometimes do this too. There is an excellent five-minute TED video available online called 'What Is Dyslexia?' by Kelli Sandman-Hurley,[9] which clearly and graphically explains the working of the dyslexic brain and the literacy problem. Recent research rightly claims that dyslexia is a phonological processing disorder, that is, a problem with being able to break a word down into separate speech sounds and then associate each of those sounds with the letters that make up the word. In other words, the problem is not with 'seeing' the word correctly but with dissecting and manipulating the component parts of the word to make sense of it.

For all reading tasks the words need to be broken down and for all spelling tasks the words need to be built up – each word has to be attacked sound by sound, rule by rule, syllable by syllable. Students who don't know how to do this or who find this difficult to do will not be able to unlock the mystery that is literacy.

The expectation that each student must learn thousands of words both by sight and off by heart is just not viable or practicable for students with a specific learning difficulty and does not take account of the fact that many also have poor memory skills. Without the proper tools students with these difficulties can spend an inordinate amount of time trying to break down each word. This is made more difficult for them because the

English language is a hybrid language with many diverse rules and influences involving words imported from other languages. To make matters worse, there is then a domino effect because slow laborious reading has a negative impact on their reading comprehension, which in turn makes reading a distressing rather than a pleasurable task. It is a case of the harder it is the harder it gets; one problem creates another and all together they make life very difficult for the person with dyslexia. Additionally, some dyslexic students will spell words phonetically; this means the word will sound correct but will be misspelt because a particular rule either wasn't known or hadn't been applied. Examples of this would be spelling 'sik' for 'sick' or 'fone' for 'phone'.

The way to help is – instead of doing more of the same that does not work – each student needs a systematic hierarchical approach that goes right back to the beginning. This means starting at a pre-reading and pre-spelling stage of literacy by providing auditory (hearing), visual (seeing) and orally tactile or oral kinaesthetic feedback, which means using the *feeling* of how a sound is made coming from how you shape or place the tongue, teeth and lips to make a particular sound. This is an intrinsic part of a speech and language therapist's work and intervention. This way the student can apply their preferred learning method (modality) to recognise the letter symbols that match the speech sound or phoneme required. I am acutely aware that some teaching methods involve a kinaesthetic (touch) approach using sandpaper letters or something similar for learning sounds, but this abrasive tactile feedback can be problematic for some dyslexic students, because the physical reaction can be similar to that of the sound of squeaky chalk or fingernails scraping on a blackboard.

Remediation is about training and retraining the brain. The approach must integrate the functions of the left and right sides (or hemispheres) of the brain. This is so that the brain can be retrained to recognise the written word. Think of the right hemisphere of the brain as that of the artist, where it deals with imagination, creativity, humour, colour and drawings. The left hemisphere is like that of the accountant: factual, analytical and linear, dealing with letters, numbers and formulas. Successful literacy programmes will draw on the skills from both sides or hemispheres, left and right. The left side lets the student analyse words and apply any rules being taught. The right side lets the student memorise unusual spellings and visualise or make mental movies of the information heard or read so that it can be readily understood and remembered. It gets all the brain involved in solving the problem creatively.

An effective literacy programme should have the following components:

- It should use phonemes (speech sounds) rather than phonetics (letter names), which is the standard approach used by speech and language therapists. Recent research in this area suggests using a phonemic rather than a phonetic approach for teaching literacy skills, which is now being adopted in more and more schools in Ireland. It works like this:
  - The word 'car' has three letters, each with their own phonetic sound: /c – a – r/
  - However, the word 'car' has only two speech sounds or phonemes: /c – ar/

  When using the phonetic approach with letter sounds, quite often the combination of the individual letter names doesn't make sense to a student. Recently I assessed an eight-year-old child with severe reading difficulties, who tackled even simple words using the 'letter sound' by 'letter sound' approach, e.g. when reading the word 'her' she broke it down into three individual letter sounds as /h – e – ru/.

Try voicing the sounds yourself: it's no wonder the child was bewildered!

- No matter what age the student is, the programme should start from the very beginning, i.e. at the pre-reading and pre-spelling stage of literacy development. It should explain that although there are 26 letters in the English alphabet, it is generally accepted that there are 44 speech sounds in the English language. Right from the start, if a student doesn't learn and know how these sounds are read or written they will almost certainly have a reading and spelling difficulty. The programme should use vowel and consonant charts to demonstrate and explain these sounds. These charts become the bedrock of their literacy development. The charts should be used to let the student see, for example, that the sound /ae/ can be written as 'a', 'ae', 'ai', 'ay', 'ei' or 'eigh' in words like acorn, ate, aid, bay, vein and eight. They will also learn to recognise when and where these various sounds should be used in a word. Without this basic knowledge all students will struggle when trying to read or spell unfamiliar words.

- Once the individual speech sounds and their various letter representations are known the student should then learn to read and spell one-syllable nonsense words (sometimes called pseudo-words) that will improve their word attack skills. The reason for using nonsense words is to stop the student recognising or guessing at familiar words. This forces them to use the newly learned sound–symbol links that are taught using the vowel and consonant charts. From an assessment perspective, I see a large number of students whose overall reading score is down primarily because of the low score they achieved in the pseudo-word naming subsection in the WIAT-II attainment test for reading. This test is administered by a psychologist. If students are not taught a specific skill they cannot be expected to be proficient at it.

- Basic reading and spelling rules should be taught in detail, with exercises to consolidate what has been taught. At this stage in my WordsWorthLearning programme, I teach twenty core rules. An example of one of these rules is the 'c/k/s' (or /-c/, /-k/ or /-ck/) rule. This rule teaches the student things like:

  - When to write a 'c' rather than a 'k' in a word, e.g. cat versus kit
  - When to write / -ck/ in a word rather than just 'c' or 'k', e.g. back versus bake
  - When to write a 'c' or a 'k' at the end of a word, e.g. park versus panic
  - Why the word 'cake' uses both a 'c' and a 'k' in its spelling
  - When to choose a 'c' over an 's' in a word, e.g. decide versus beside
  - When to write /-ss/, /-ce/, /-se/ or /-ze/ endings in a word, e.g. miss, rice, rise or blaze

  Over many years I have been able to work out a consistent formula to explain such rules. Interestingly, at a recent British Educational Training and Technology (BETT) show in London, I asked some of my competitors about their approach to the c/k/s rule and the answer was to provide long lists of words that had these letter combinations that the student had to learn off by heart. Nothing new there! My approach is to provide one formula that applies to thousands of words, rather than providing thousands of words to learn off by heart without any logical explanation.

- The next stage in literacy intervention should involve introducing basic single-syllable real words for reading and spelling that incorporate and consolidate the rules and theories that were previously taught. These words should be taught in three stages: firstly introduce words that have a direct sound–symbol association where no rule is utilised, e.g. 'pot'; the next stage should introduce words that incorporate the more common and troublesome rules, for example with the c/k/s rule words like cake, kite, back, dark, cent, sent, scent, miss, rice and rise should be introduced and the reason for each pattern explained; and the final stage should focus on complex words that incorporate more irregular or foreign-language-influenced rules, e.g. why /ch/ is a /k/ sound in some words like 'ache' or 'school'. In my clinical opinion, at this stage it is too early to introduce words with two or more syllables because the student needs to understand syllable division rules first. I believe current school practice is to provide a variety of single-syllable and multi-syllabic words if they rhyme with or contain a particular sound that is the topic of the lesson, for example '**know**', '**know**ledge', 'ac**know**ledge'. I believe this practice is inappropriate without provision of the reasons and tools for syllabication beforehand. To me this puts the cart before the horse and unfortunately it sets a dyslexic student up to fail. Similarly, using wordlists like the Dolch list for spelling, without teaching basic sound and rule knowledge, puts the emphasis on memory, which for many people with dyslexia is their point of failure. For some complex words or, as I like to call them, 'outlaws' (because they have no rules), something else is required. Students need a colourful and coded visualisation technique to help anchor the word image in long-term memory. We often remember what we see, especially if it is visually attractive. Visual hooks are extremely important and many of the rules that I have developed and retrofitted for the English language explain these outlaws with a visual component to reinforce the idea and aid memory.

- When the basic single-syllable words have been conquered the next stage should be an introduction to syllable division rules that should be taught for both reading and spelling.

Syllable division rules are strategies that teach how to know where to split a word into its individual syllables or beats; it is the rhythm of the word. For example, 'car' has one syllable or beat, 'car-pet' has two and 'car-a-van' has three, and so on. I teach nine syllable division rules for both reading and spelling. You should find out from your child's teacher what is being used in their school to teach syllable division rules, because some of the rules that are used in current 'reading only' programmes actually distort spelling. An example of this occurs in one widely used learning support reading programme in Irish schools, where the programme teaches that when there is a vowel-consonant-consonant-vowel (VCCV) combination in a word, the word should be split after the second consonant, e.g. **traff/ic**. Whereas this approach certainly works for reading, in my opinion it distorts spelling. When spelling words such as 'traffic' with the VCCV combination, you should always stop before the double consonant, i.e. 'tra/ffic'. The reason for this is that when a syllable or beat ends in a *short vowel* (/a, e, i, o, u/) you must always double the next consonant letter. Although you only hear one 'f' in traffic, you must write two. From a clinical perspective, I often see students who have already been through the mill and have tried a variety of literacy remedial programmes that have produced little or no academic gain. My initial intervention begins with helping the student to *unlearn* misleading rules before I can teach them rules that actually *do* work.

- The next stage should focus on developing an in-depth knowledge of prefixes (for example 'un' in unhappy), suffixes (for example 'ing' in talking) and common word endings (such as 'ive' in active). These should also include influences from foreign languages that have been integrated into the English language. Endings originating from French (e.g. -ique), Latin (e.g. -tion) or Greek (e.g. -ism) in particular should be explained in full. An example: how do you know when to write the ending /-cian/ instead of /-tian/, in words like 'magician' or 'Martian'?

- Sequencing (the order of letters and sounds in a word), left–right orientation (which is not just knowing your left from right but also understanding that English script is read or written from the left-hand side of the page, line or word), auditory discrimination (the ability to hear and tell the difference between sounds, e.g. /p/ from /b/), and memory skills are integral parts of any literacy programme and should be taught and embedded within the literacy tasks.

- Reading and spelling skills are on the oral-language–literate continuum, by which I mean that they are an extension of your oral language development (how you speak) into written language (how you read and write the written word); the emphasis should be placed on vocabulary enrichment (learning new words) with overall language stimulation throughout. As mentioned in previous chapters, students with literacy difficulties will usually have associated language deficits as well, which are evident when a student demonstrates a poor vocabulary repertoire or knowledge, has difficulty following instructions or finds it hard to express what they want to say, particularly when under pressure.

Having conducted many language assessments over the years, one observation that is particularly interesting is that students with literacy difficulties also tend to have a poorer vocabulary range. As you might expect, this is mainly due to the lack of exposure to words because they don't read for enjoyment and so don't come across as many new words as children who do. If a child's reading level is below their actual age they will only be able to read books written for a younger age group and as a consequence they are only exposed to immature language in general. This puts them at a disadvantage in their age group. This can be remediated using a programme that puts a heavy emphasis on vocabulary development. Students not only improve their literacy skills but also simultaneously improve their language skills. Over my years as a speech and language therapist I have been fascinated with the benefits of changing the focus of therapy – this is because I understand dyslexia as someone who has it. I work through literacy to promote language skills, which is the opposite strategy to that taken with the more traditional approach.

- A good programme should contain enough rules and formulas that will cover most of the words in the English language, although there will always be a few outlaws (complex words that don't follow the rules). If the student isn't taught to use rules then they will have to rely on memory skills, which can be a major hurdle because memory problems often go hand-in-hand with dyslexia. The formulas and rules become automatic with regular practice or drill and enter the student's subconscious, much like learning to drive a car. You start by learning the *Rules of the Road* and then how to operate and drive the car. As a competent driver how often do you have to stop and think about all the manoeuvres required to get you from A to B? Probably never: this is the ultimate aim when using this type of literacy intervention.

- To really engage today's children, literacy programmes need to at least have an online component, with video tutorials and graphical interactive exercises. This way, students can access all the instruction and information they need through a medium they feel comfortable with and probably use every day. This normalises learning for them and makes it fun. For learning, an additional benefit is that students can replay instructional video tutorials as often as they like if they missed a bit or didn't fully understand the concept being taught first time around. The interactive exercises can also be replayed to allow the student to try out and consolidate the information that has been taught. This also allows them to learn at their own pace and in their own time.

- To keep the students motivated they need to be able to track their progress so that they know where they currently are in the programme and how much they have still to do to finish it. Without this information learning can feel like an endless, draining task. Your child's teacher will have lesson plans, which they can share in a simple format with their students so they know what to do and what their goals are. Recently, after taking advice from parents and children who were using our programme, we incorporated progress bars for each of the tutorials and exercises, which has been a resounding success. Apparently it has really motivated the students to proceed and complete each task in hand and reach the end of the programme. It is hugely motivating to track your own progress and then to set the goal of getting to the end of the progress bar.
- Effective programmes will also have ongoing evaluation of progress or informal testing throughout the programme, so that a teacher or parent can identify any items that need to be revised and reinforced before moving on to the next level.
- Ideally the programme should be designed to be used both at home and in school, without the need for any formal training. This will allow a collaborative approach between the parent, teacher and student where they can all be involved in working together to improve the student's learning and progress.
- All interventions should have a proven track record with measurable results. Be wary of suppliers that provide only

anecdotal evidence that their products work. You should look for confirmed evidence-based or results-based evidence before proceeding.

Finally, don't be afraid to move from the old methods to embark on new – but tried, tested and proven – approaches for, as in the words of Francis Bacon, 'if we are to achieve things never before accomplished we must employ methods never before attempted.'

* * *

We live in a world where products make promises. Not everything does what it says on the tin. This chapter discusses some of the many remedial products, services and approaches on offer in the marketplace today that claim to work miracles, without clear evidence of their effectiveness.

It also covers in detail what, as a clinician, is my preferred therapy approach for learning competent reading and spelling skills. I believe the evidence and outcomes of this remedial process suggests that it is the method that works best for dyslexia and reading and/or spelling disorders.

Having read this chapter, the reader will have a better understanding of the best approach to remediate a specific learning difficulty, including dyslexia.

7

WORKING TOGETHER: HOME, SCHOOL AND OTHERS

Up to the point of being approached to write this book I was of the opinion that very little in life could genuinely surprise me – I was totally wrong. Firstly, I was flabbergasted to be asked to write a book about dyslexia because the whole thought of writing something of that scale fed into my every dread. Secondly, it was a revelation to me that someone who actually knew me and was aware of my dyslexic background would even think that I would be able to do it.

The genesis of this book evolved from a meeting with clinical psychologist and writer Dr Marie Murray, which turned out to be quite a story: we met for lunch in early January 2014 where she proposed the idea that I might write a book about my personal and clinical experience of dyslexia. She believed that my life experiences, my professional training, my years of practice and my WordsWorthLearning programme should be narrated in book form. She thought that it was important to let every person with dyslexia know that they can succeed, even in things they believe to be impossible. I was swept away by her wonderful enthusiasm, belief and persuasion that I could actually take this on. Although it seemed at first to be a mammoth challenge, my fears were assuaged when she assured me that I would be guided through this unknown territory and process.

All through lunch my stomach churned, contracted and revolted, which I thought was simply a reaction to my fear and anxiety. However, I was determined that I was going to overcome it. After a long lunch we parted ways and went home. A couple of hours later the root cause of my nausea became clear when I ended up in hospital for what turned out to be an emergency appendectomy! While lying for most of the night on a trolley in the corridor, I was diverted from any thoughts of pain by sheer panic about what I had agreed to do. That's what it's like having dyslexia: the anxiety is lifelong. The doubts crept in and I started questioning myself. Could I do it? Would it be any good? More importantly, would anyone want to read it?

Only you, the reader, can answer the last two questions but I can now answer the first question because, to my huge surprise, I have proven to myself that I can write a book. Yes, I can write a book and my dyslexia actually helped me to do it. Of course, a key factor that helped me through the process to complete the task was the clear direction and guidance from Marie, without which I might still be looking at a blank page. Never underestimate the value of informed, reliable advice and direction to guide you through unknown territory.

Something that surprised me to an extent during the course of writing this book was that it became more and more apparent to me just how many of the things about dyslexia that I've taken for granted over the years are not generally known or understood. On reflection, I realised that my combined personal and professional experience of dyslexia gave me a much deeper insight and also that I had a wealth of information about dyslexia that others, perhaps, don't have. I began to realise how quickly I recognised clear indicators of dyslexia and, for the most part, my ability to identify a correct prognosis for each individual child. I seem to know instinctively what each child needs to do to succeed. During my career I have also discovered that:

- There is NO reliable group assessment test for reading accuracy (the mechanics of reading) available worldwide; there are many good tests that can be administered individually, but none for a group. That means group reading tests such as the Drumcondra or the MICRA-T, which are being used in schools in Ireland today, do not test how well your child is actually reading, they only test for:
  ○ Vocabulary knowledge
  ○ Reading comprehension, or how much is understood when reading silently
  These are two very different tasks to that of testing for the mechanics of reading.
- Although there are very good group spelling tests available, my experience is that many schools in Ireland don't formally test spelling with a standardised test. Consequently, there are no accurate national statistics available for students who present with spelling difficulties. The dreaded class spelling test (normally on a Friday) only demonstrates short-term memory ability. Children with problems like dyslexia can quickly forget words they have learned by heart for the spelling test, because they haven't been anchored in long-term memory.
- Many parents have expressed difficulty understanding the professional jargon used in formal assessment reports. It's a bit like *Goldilocks and the Three Bears*: some reports have too much technical wording that just confuses the reader, some are so scant they carry very little useful information, and some are 'just right', giving a clear definition and direction. As professionals, we all need to review and revise our report writing to ensure the reports are accessible and understandable to the readers. This, in turn, will empower the recipient to follow the right path when taking things to the next stage.
- Unfortunately, at this time, too few psychologists, teachers, occupational therapists or indeed speech and language

therapists are aware of the importance of the role that a speech and language therapist (SLT) can play in remediating dyslexia or any other reading or spelling disorder. The SLT assessment can delve deeper into some of the broader elements on the oral–literate continuum identified in the earlier reports from other professionals and can recommend and provide a suitable therapy process to achieve a positive outcome. These recommendations are crucial.

- Over the years I've received many psychological assessment reports that contain a long list of recommendations for interventions that might be considered. However, because these reports are often not informed by the specific detail of the SLT assessment, they may lack a hierarchy in their recommendations for the specific child. While the recommendations provided in such reports may have generic merit, because they are not specifically designed for the individual child they may be contraindicated for a particular child.

- Additionally, it can be inadvisable for the recommendations to be implemented simultaneously. On occasion, they can even contradict or cancel each other out or in some cases they might not be warranted at all. It is, therefore, important that you work with your child using a specific, individually designed recommendation list to be implemented with your child at their pace.

- Another area of concern is that the benefit of professionals working together in a multidisciplinary environment, i.e. sharing and communicating ideas and advice about a client/child, particularly in a school setting, can be insufficiently recognised. Without those multidisciplinary interactions there is a danger of individual professionals becoming too entrenched in the ideologies of their own disciplines or professions, uninformed by the value of shared perspectives which enhance the work for everyone. I'm often asked by parents to contact a psychologist or teacher, or both, in order to clarify a point, and for the benefit of everyone we professionals should connect more often to consider the most appropriate intervention path for the client/child concerned. A coordinated and collaborative plan has to be best for the child.

- Too often, parents don't actually know precisely what materials or method is being used in 'learning support' or 'resource' classes at school. Although most will know how many sessions have been sanctioned and whether or not the remedial work is in a group or on a one-to-one basis, it's very rare that a parent will know exactly what materials are being used and what the individual approach and projected learning outcomes will be. Additionally, many parents don't know how they can meaningfully, at home with their child, support the literacy intervention being used in learning support. It's worth contacting your child's teacher to find out what programme or materials are being used with a view to seeking specific instructions on how to help to generalise and consolidate the work at home.

- Parents are now expecting more collaboration between home, school and/or therapists. They are right to do so. We need to share information and observations and give feedback about progress or lack of progress. The more school visits I do the more I realise how beneficial they are for everyone, including myself, in trying to help the child. The only drawback is the difficulty in coordinating a timetable that is suitable for all who need to attend, taking into account everyone's busy schedules.

- My advice to parents is to ask each of the professionals involved the following:
  ○ What questions should I be asking to get a greater understanding of my child's position?

○ If this was your child what additional information would you want to know?

○ What further investigations would you consider appropriate?

○ What signs should I be looking out for that I haven't already mentioned or possibly haven't noticed?

If there are some signs brought to your attention, then ask:

○ What should I do now to deal with these additional observations?

○ Over and above supervising any homework, what else can I do to support what is being taught in the classroom?

Parents want feedback and want to be included, they want to get involved and they can make a valuable contribution to the total educational process.

I recently came across a very interesting infographic of a study sourced from the US Department of Education.[10] The study showed the effects that parental involvement had on a student's academic performance. There were four interesting facts reported:

- Students who were taught to recognise all their letters, could count to twenty, could write their first name and were read to on a nightly basis prior to starting primary school went on to achieve advanced third-level degrees.
- Students from families where there was less tutoring at home and little school collaboration were more likely to repeat a year in primary school.
- Students enjoyed school more when their parents worked collaboratively with the school.
- Students achieved higher grades in general when their parents worked collaboratively with the school.

From an Irish perspective, a study by Eivers and Creaven[11] reported that:

- 69 per cent of Irish parents helped their child with their homework on a daily or almost daily basis.
- Irish principals and teachers were extremely positive about parental support for pupil achievement and parental involvement in school activities.
- Irish teachers were well below average in the frequency with which they had parent–teacher meetings to discuss students' progress.
- Irish schools were far less likely to give regular parental updates on the behaviour and well-being of students.
- Irish schools were less likely to discuss parental concerns or wishes about their child's learning and progress.

Unfortunately, the study results above are very similar to the reports and comments that I get from parents. Without clear and frequent communication between the multi-disciplines and parents, many important issues are either missed or never dealt with.

Although this might appear to be critical of schools and teachers, I have the greatest respect for teachers, having worked in schools and also in close collaboration with teachers over many years during my career. With that experience, I fully appreciate the huge demands and constraints placed on educators, with ever-changing policies, funding and resource problems, and an ever-expanding curriculum to be met. Nevertheless, I believe it is now time for all professionals working in the education sector to become more creative in the delivery of their services in a multidisciplinary fashion. It is much easier today for people to communicate using internet technology and very few don't have access to devices such as a PC, tablet or even mobile devices.

I recently became aware of and quite excited about an ingenious concept that has been gathering momentum in the education sector in the United States over the last ten years. With the convergence of faster broadband and video streaming it has become more common for schools to use that technology to record lessons and make them available to the students online. It is called the 'flipped classroom' model. To explain, it involves creating and providing lessons online, thus moving them out of the classroom and allowing each student to view the lesson content in their own time, at their own pace and in their preferred environment. This approach is certainly not a replacement for good quality classroom-based teaching; however, it gives the student more opportunity to reflect on what they are learning and the added benefit is that they can also rewind and review tutorials that they may have found challenging. They can do this as often as they like, providing the opportunity to work at their own pace. This is crucial for dyslexic students for whom repetition and reinforcement are often necessary to understand complex concepts. In the classroom, teachers can then determine more accurately who has grasped what and crucially which areas will require reinforcement. It gives the teacher a clearer idea and more focused time with individual students to consolidate the lesson and provide a greater opportunity for questions and discussion to develop a deeper understanding of what is being taught. It also allows for the integration of additional supportive materials that might suit certain individuals' learning styles, e.g. mind maps, graphs or mnemonics (memory aids). A good recent example of using a mnemonic to aid memory was when I was working with a seventeen-year-old who was studying the Irish 1916 Easter Rising and she was having difficulty remembering the names of the main leaders (as was I, I might add), so I quickly worked out this formula: PMC PMC + C (**P**earse, **M**acDiarmada, **C**larke, **P**lunkett,

MacDonagh, Ceannt and Connolly). This is now another formula firmly embedded in both of our memories. The flipped classroom model also provides a better platform for encouraging collaborative or group activities in the class and this has a real benefit for those who need a little more time to absorb and understand the lesson.

To explain a bit further: traditionally the role of the teacher is to give lessons in class and set homework for the new information to be reinforced at home. There are many problems with this traditional approach, such as:

- Students learn at different speeds; some grasp concepts quickly while others need more time to process new ideas.
- Attention span can wander for some, with important pieces of information being missed. (These lapses of attention tend to be more common with students who are struggling.)
- When a student misses a class, which can be for a number of reasons, e.g. sports or illness, they can miss out on a lot of important information that may not be repeated at a later stage.
- When doing homework, students may not remember what or how they were taught to do something, so get stuck. Many report that they were unable to transcribe their homework down from the board correctly or quickly enough – this is a common occurrence with dyslexic and dyspraxic students. I was recently working with a dyspraxic and dyslexic boy, who because of his difficulties is allowed to transcribe history notes from the teacher's PowerPoint presentation onto his iPad in class. He was studying the Renaissance but later couldn't make sense of his notes as he had misspelled so many of the key words that his errors distorted his comprehension of the facts; for example, instead of writing 'artists'

patrons', he had written *'patriots'*, which set him off on a totally different tangent.

- Struggling students must proceed at the same speed as the class, so don't have personal time to rationalise what they have been taught. Consequently, they don't fully understand it.
- Quite often if a student doesn't understand a new concept in class they don't want to draw attention to their confusion and as a result they never get the chance to fully understand the concept and it gets missed.

The benefits of the flipped classroom approach are multiple:

- Parents are given clear directions, a work schedule and materials to use with their child at home.
- The students are set certain video tutorials to watch at home, along with engaging interactive exercises. A student can pause, rewind and replay any of the lessons at any time, so they can genuinely learn at their own pace in a less stressed environment.
- Discussing the course work at home gives the parent a much clearer picture of their child's understanding of the concepts being taught at school and alerts them to what additional help or reinforcement they may need.
- Discussing the homework in the classroom gives the teacher a much clearer focus concerning those students who 'get it' and those who need a bit more help.
- Homework is discussed with the whole class, which allows all students to develop a deeper understanding of what is being taught. It also facilitates peer tuition and support, which I have always found to be a very powerful teaching tool in therapy.

- The teacher can also introduce additional materials to support, consolidate and expand on what is being taught.
- It promotes a 'learning together' ethos where all students participate in class and help each other and at home parents can participate and collaborate with the teachers.
- It empowers students and parents to take responsibility for their learning and allows them more freedom to experiment and explore.

As with all good ideas, there are some difficulties or drawbacks and clearly this approach would take some time to establish across the education sector, given the radical changes required. In the shorter term, there are ready-made programmes that could be used with this model that provide a creative solution for those students with specific learning difficulties who are in need of additional remedial support. For example, some schools are using the WordsWorthLearning programme as a pilot flipped classroom model for struggling students, with extremely encouraging results.

One case study to demonstrate the effectiveness of this approach is that of 'Sarah', a ten-year-old girl whose reading and spelling skills were initially assessed by her learning support teacher. On the Neale Analysis of Reading Ability II, Sarah's reading accuracy skills were 26 months behind her chronological age (actual age), her reading comprehension score was 24 months behind and her spelling, as tested on the Vernon Graded Word Spelling Test, was 56 months behind her actual age. Because one of her scores (her spelling) gave her a percentile ranking of at or below the 10th percentile for her age, she was eligible for learning support for spelling, but she was clearly underperforming on reading tasks too. As a result, she was chosen to be one of eight children to participate in the flipped classroom project within her school. This project ran for five months, with her parents working collaboratively with the learning support teacher. Daily tasks were set to complete online at home and then the students were seen in a group session once a week in school to revise and support the focused concepts initially taught at home. After the five months Sarah was reassessed by the learning support teacher to evaluate her progress. As five months has lapsed it would be expected that Sarah would have made five months' progress on re-testing. Over the five months Sarah's reading accuracy skills improved by eighteen months, her reading comprehension improved by ten months and her spelling improved by a whopping thirty-seven months. This profile of success is not unusual with or specific to the pilot study group; in fact this accelerated level of improvement has become the norm rather than the exception for students who undergo this effective approach to intervention.

The whole complex area of specific learning difficulty, with its many associated difficulties for some, is a minefield even though it is also a well-trodden path. Without fail, every time I mention what I do professionally someone in the group either has direct experience of a specific learning difficulty or knows someone with this difficulty. If your child is experiencing difficulty you are not alone. What is important though is to do something about it as soon as it is flagged. While it is never too late to treat a specific learning difficulty, the longer it is left unattended to the more complicated it becomes. Talk openly about your concerns because invariably you will come across someone who has already gone through the process and who will be able to advise you on the best route possible while at the same time warning you about the hidden pitfalls. Help is available so do look for it as soon as possible.

***

This chapter highlights the following:

- Collaboration between parents and professionals is the key to success.
- Professional reports need to be clear and client-friendly.
- It is important to understand the recommendations given, why they are being recommended, the order in which they should be carried out and the reasons why not all will be necessary. In other words, depending on the therapeutic route you choose to take, only some of the recommendations would be required. So seek clarification from the assessor on this at the time of receiving the report.
- The benefits of the flipped classroom model for students who are struggling, including those who are not eligible for learning support
- The importance of talking openly about your child's dyslexia, as it is very common problem

8

EMOTIONAL IMPACT: EMBARRASSMENT AND SHAME

Most of us have a deep desire to 'fit in'; particularly when we are children we just want to be the same as everyone else. In situations where we are not the same, where we can't fit in, communicate in the same way as other people, keep up at school, be as good as the next person at sports, get chosen for a team, manage riding a bike or kicking a football, playing tennis or swimming or running without falling, it is distressing. It is important not to be clumsy when you are a child, to be able to see, to hear what is going on, to be able to take homework down and do it, to get changed quickly after sport, to understand jokes, to be able to communicate effectively and to know what is going on and be part of it. In any situation where we feel different and don't want to be different, then it damages our confidence. We can feel embarrassed, humbled, humiliated and even ashamed when we are different. We can feel that we are not 'normal'. We can feel abnormal.

So, what is normal? Who determines what is normal and who has the right to make anyone feel abnormal? I don't have the answers to these questions, but from an early age, having lived with undiagnosed dyslexia, I have experienced most of the difficulties of being different first-hand, especially the feeling of being ashamed. No person, let alone a child, should have to go through that experience, and it is something that really needs to be recognised and addressed.

In all probability, we all know someone who has one or more common disorders such as dyslexia, dyspraxia, dysgraphia or ADHD, to name but a few. These conditions are present for many people we come across in our day-to-day living and thankfully these conditions are understood better now and they have, for the most part, lost their stigma. Having said that, even today the mention of dyslexia can still be shrouded with shame and embarrassment and at times it seems that the false antiquated notion still exists that dyslexia equates with stupidity. Most people are willing to disclose that they suffer from common disorders like migraine, asthma, diabetes or eczema, but rarely will they disclose that they are dyslexic, unless they have been through successful intervention or have received positive and balanced support in both home and academic settings.

The lengths some people will go to to hide or disguise the fact that they have or their child has dyslexia are remarkable. This often masks other associated difficulties, yet if the problem had been addressed from the start, from when it was first noticed, then it might never have developed and caused the subsequent emotional damage that it can do. From a clinical perspective I find it interesting but by no means a coincidence that problems escalate and compounding issues tend to occur at three key stages:

- Around eight years of age
- Around thirteen years of age – heading into the adolescent years
- In or around eighteen years of age – heading into young adulthood

The Childhood Years

By eight years of age a student will most likely be in second class, having completed three formal primary school grades. If their reading and spelling skills are lagging behind their classmates they will already be acutely aware of that difference. Depending on the severity, they may be leaving the class to attend learning support, probably on a daily basis. For many this 'streaming' is in itself a cause for embarrassment, unless it is handled sensitively both in school and at home. Some of the parents who attend my clinics request that I don't mention or use the 'dyslexia' label in front of their child. Essentially, they want to hide the fact that there is a problem from their child. I make a point of being clinically correct and I am always sensitive to each family's needs and requests. That being said, however, every child who attends my practice is fully aware that they are attending for a reason. If that reason is not disclosed it can add to the child's anxiety. With this in mind, I do recommend that parents talk openly and frankly to their child in age-appropriate language and explain their goal in bringing their child to me so that the child understands the concern and the proposed solution. In this way I believe that the child's anxieties are allayed. In my own experience, the unknown is far more terrifying than the known.

There is no doubt that some parents actively avoid the use of the dyslexia label and somehow view it as something to be ashamed of and concealed. This tends to arise from parents' natural inherent protectiveness and their understandable wish not to have their child feel different in any way. My aim is to help parents to see that their child simply has a different way of learning that requires support, validation and acceptance because the essence of dyslexia is a different way of viewing not only written language but the world in general – and others need to be aware of that. It involves a different way of thinking, of understanding and of problem-solving to that which is deemed to be the norm. This difference can often be a positive characteristic, which when nurtured can open up a totally new creative world and future for the child. Tragically, it can, for some, take a lifetime of self-doubt before recognising and coming to terms with its existence. Children who are dyslexic know that they are different and by not acknowledging and embracing this difference it can make the situation worse for the child. Clinically, I find that when a child comes to understand that the problem they are experiencing has a specific name and can be partially, if not totally, resolved in many cases that child's relief is palpable.

When young children become aware that they are under-performing academically this can lead to many associated problems, such as:

- Signs of anxiety, e.g. nail biting, avoiding social situations and school avoidance
- Comfort eating
- Becoming socially isolated – not engaging in playground games where the rules can vary, causing confusion for the child
- Showing mild psychosomatic complaints such as a sore tummy or headache on school days
- Showing an unusual clinginess, which is not displayed in non-academic settings
- Bedwetting, again only happening during school terms
- Extreme fatigue – needing much more sleep than their siblings or peers
- Showing outbursts of anger or getting upset without any apparent reason or cause
- Being bullied or involved in bullying other children they might consider to be inferior to themselves

These signs, although they might not be overly severe, are classic cries for help from a child and they should be heeded. The list above is not an exhaustive one but if you notice your child is showing any other signs of distress you should investigate immediately and deal with the underlying cause. Hiding from, ignoring or disguising a problem doesn't make it go away; it will only make it worse for your child over time.

The Teenage or Adolescent Years

By thirteen years of age, students naturally have to contend with the onset of puberty and the turmoil of adolescence but if, on top of that, they have a specific learning difficulty like dyslexia, they will also have to deal with the significant increase in academic demands that occur at secondary level education without the capacity to meet them. Reading stops being a 'subject' in secondary school and becomes a means to an end, a way of gaining information, studying a topic and learning. Poor academic success can trigger low self-esteem, frustration, avoidance and, in some cases, 'acting out'. There is a recognised relationship between emotional and/or behavioural difficulties and specific learning and language difficulties. This is not new and has been documented in research studies over many decades, but it often gets forgotten and the focus can be on the young person's behaviour as the primary problem while forgetting that there may be an underlying academic struggle going on.

Many adolescents with language and literacy difficulties can also experience associated difficulties with social relationships and emotional health. Common symptoms include low self-esteem, poor self-image, depression and anxiety. Students who have undiagnosed and/or untreated specific learning difficulties can also show an increase in behavioural problems that may appear to be attention or concentration difficulties, ADHD, conduct disorders or anti-social behaviours. This can first become apparent during the mid- to late years in primary school and onwards into adolescence.

It is well documented that boys and girls with specific learning difficulties tend to display their feelings differently. Boys tend to present with externalised obvious symptoms such as conduct or behaviour disorders, which are an attempt to distract from their underlying academic difficulties by bringing attention to bad behaviour, or hiding their academic problems by becoming the class clown. Girls, on the other hand, tend to demonstrate more internalised or hidden distress and have an inferior academic self-image; in other words, they rate themselves lower in academic domains than their peers, exhibiting negative self-beliefs. Their own internal dialogue reinforces their belief that they can't do the task or can't achieve even if they try, which for many isn't actually the case. They often try to stay under the radar in the hope of going unnoticed, their rationale being that if they don't bring attention to themselves they won't be found out – right? These girls tend towards higher incidences of anxiety and minor psychosomatic complaints than their classmates who are not experiencing academic difficulties. In more extreme situations, girls can show higher rates of depression, incidences of self-harming and suicidal ideation, and in extreme situations be at suicidal risk. As they get older, if the academic challenges are not properly addressed both boys and girls tend to have high rates of school avoidance, truanting, early school-leaving and in extreme cases some may even engage in more serious delinquent behaviours.

Emotional and behavioural problems can often be secondary to the specific learning difficulty. Many years ago, while I was the principal speech and language therapist in a child and adolescent mental health service (CAMHS), working as part of a multidisciplinary team, I was asked to conduct language and literacy assessments on all the child and adolescent inpatients who were in the onsite residential unit. This unit, which no longer exists, was set up for young people with serious emotional and/or behavioural difficulties. Although this unit was additional to my normal clinical workload, I was very interested in participating in this research as I was aware that some of the children referred in with difficulties such as eating disorders, school refusal, self-harming, depression or suicidal ideation had undiagnosed underlying language and/or literacy difficulties. While I don't remember the exact number of children who were resident at the time, what has always stayed in my mind is that every single child in residence at that point had a significant language and/or literacy difficulty that was compounding or complicating their situation. Of course, for me this raises the 'chicken and egg' question: which came first? Was the specific learning difficulty the root cause of their problems or was it just another area of deficit to contend with? Whatever the answer, it demonstrably highlighted the need for a multidisciplinary approach to both learning difficulties and emotional distress with all relevant professions working in tandem as one team.

The Adult Years

Adulthood brings with it additional challenges for anyone on the 'journey of shame' in terms of social, family, study and work responsibilities. The pressure is always there to appear normal and confident, with no outward signs of having a difficulty or anything that might expose the inner turmoil. Feelings of inferiority, insecurity and frustration persist into adulthood. The inferiority complex and inherent shame is well-cemented and it becomes more and more difficult to shed that mantle.

Adults with untreated reading and spelling disorders or dyslexia tend to avoid all situations that might expose their secret.

I clearly remember an incident that occurred in my final year in college. I always had an interest in stuttering or dysfluency and an opportunity arose for final-year speech and language therapy students to volunteer to get involved in a therapy project with adult stutterers. I was fascinated by the prospect and saw it as a great opportunity to learn about the area, as I knew I would learn much more by implementing the intervention skills I was being taught rather than reading about how to do it. Without hesitation I put my name forward, only to withdraw it some days later. It had come to my attention that as one of the student therapists I may at times have to read aloud to the group, which for me was an absolute no-no. The senior lecturer involved with the project, to my knowledge, was unaware of my dyslexia and I had no intention of informing her – my shame and embarrassment at my difficulties at the time was so great. Having weighed up the options it was preferable to me to be perceived as disinterested or unreliable rather than stupid. Thinking back to that time and the choice I made still bothers me today. It bothers me on behalf of others too, who might lose out on opportunities they would love to have, or be misconstrued as being disinterested, lacking motivation, lazy or lacking commitment when, in fact, they are just scared of being 'found out'. Imagine I was not able to say 'I'd love to do this but I struggle to read out loud'. So deep were the years of covering up my dyslexia and being embarrassed by it, so deeply had those years influenced me, that my fear took over and denied me a chance I really wanted to have.

Associated difficulties in adulthood appear to be more prevalent with young men than young women, as women tend towards avoiding exposure and move into less academic jobs or they may be more likely than their non-dyslexic, more 'studious' peers to have children earlier and/or become stay-at-home mothers. On the other hand, current society trends still place pressure on the male to be the main breadwinner, so the impact is perhaps felt more by young men, who are more vulnerable to unemployment or to being in unskilled jobs with low earnings and poor prospects.

In the course of my private practice I have worked with a number of adults with significant literacy problems, most of whom I would have regarded as having classic dyslexia. With the exception of only two professional women who attended for individual therapy and who also did the online WordsWorth-Learning programme, all exhibited the following profile:

- All were highly anxious and many were tearful on initial meeting and testing.
- Only their closest family (usually a spouse) knew they had a difficulty.
- All were in low- or relatively low-skilled jobs or were unemployed.
- None had formal qualifications.
- None fully completed the programme and all bar one in this group disengaged midway through therapy; the exception to the group continued to attend the sessions but did not do the more complex exercises as directed.
- All except for one woman began with a partner, friend or spouse to facilitate with the homework but gradually the supports either fell away or the client stopped their participation. This usually occurred when their need for support was greatest.
- None believed that they could really overcome their difficulties.
- As the programme became more complex, attendance was poor and more erratic.

- All displayed significant emotional factors in relation to their difficulties, describing years of shame, embarrassment, humiliation and avoidance.
- Secrecy was a strong factor; none wanted their extended family, work colleagues or employers to know they had a difficulty or that they were attending therapy. Whereas some had to disclose their difficulty in order to get time off work, it was done under strictest confidence.
- All felt that they would be ridiculed and it would damage their job prospects if they disclosed they had dyslexia and that they were receiving remedial help. In reality, those fears didn't materialise for any of them.

I find working with adults to be both intriguing and emotional. They tend to have the language to express the deep emotions felt, along with a wealth of life experiences. I remember two men in particular, both of whom gave me great insight into the problems from another perspective – perhaps it was the important male perspective. One very bright, articulate man described his dyslexia as being like a cancer: a silent killer, all-invasive, infiltrating every aspect of his personal and professional life. He described how he would constantly be on his guard not to be found out, both at home and in work. At work he described himself as the 'king of delegators'; in other words, any tasks that required literacy skills would be subtly passed on to a colleague, while he would deal with the more hands-on aspects of the job. Although his wife was aware of his difficulties his young children were not. His motivation to have his problem remediated was that he wanted to be able to read nighttime stories to his children and to help them with their homework, both of which were beyond his capacity at the time he spoke to me. Once this man reached a level of competency that allowed him to read children's books he disengaged from therapy. His personal goal was met.

The second man with whom I worked clinically was also a very bright, ambitious man, who had come from an academic family background where expectations were high and disappointments were embarrassing. This man, let's call him Brian, then in his thirties, had the full support of his wife, who was also keen to engage in the intervention. After completing secondary education, Brian undertook a number of FÁS training courses to learn a trade. He had also attempted numerous other courses, in the intervening years, but had completed none of them. He had since set up his own company and was now struggling with the administrative tasks and the paperwork was taking him an inordinate amount of time. This was, in fact, his motivation for attending remedial therapy. During his assessment it was clear to me that Brian was severely dyslexic; he could read some of the texts if he was given more time, but the effort was visibly torturous. Midway through his assessment Brian broke down and sobbed because the exposure and embarrassment was just overwhelming for him. However, the outcome of the assessment was that we agreed to work together to improve his literacy skills.

Brian started the intervention sessions, accompanied by his partner, with great enthusiasm but quite soon cancellations began to occur and by this time his partner was no longer attending the sessions, at his request. Brian was acutely embarrassed and ashamed at showing his difficulties and although he was beginning to grasp the concepts well and was progressing, he could not be convinced that he would continue to improve. In his own internal dialogue, he had totally convinced himself that he was a failure and no amount of support or earned praise could disabuse him of that notion. Finally, I received a call from him saying that he didn't have the time to devote to the remedial therapy sessions and had decided to put them on hold.

Shame – the embodiment of shame, the impact of shame – creates a very powerful and negative paralysing emotion which, once it takes a grip, is extremely difficult to overcome. From my own experience, and also working with older students with literacy difficulties, I have found that overcoming shame is just as important for successful intervention outcomes as the literacy remedial work itself. It would be prudent for all parents or guardians who might feel their own personal shame about their child's literacy difficulties to remember that this should not be projected onto the child. This will only compound the problem, making the path for any treatment much more difficult. People with a supposed specific learning difficulty like dyslexia can be taught to read and spell simply by using a different teaching approach – there is no shame in that!

***

This chapter explores the three key stages for anyone who is dyslexic, or has a specific learning difficulty. It discusses early childhood, adolescent years and the young adulthood years, covering the associated emotional and behavioural problems that can occur at these stages.

It stresses the importance of naming and embracing the difficulty, to alleviate the embarrassment and shame, with some specific cases used as typical examples.

9

Extreme Consequences: The Dangers of Undiagnosed or Untreated Dyslexia

We live in a 'literate' world. For anyone to be excluded from it is a tragedy. This can cause frustration and denial, which can seriously affect personal, social and professional development and opportunities as those who are illiterate advance through life. It takes its toll. This is most tragically evident in those whose disadvantage brings them into conflict with institutional authority, in school, in vocational situations, in the workplace, in trying to find work and especially when they find themselves in conflict with the law.

The legal system is distinguished by the precision of its language. There is no room for ambiguity, for vague, careless, slipshod, loose expression. Guilt or innocence in court may depend upon oratory, upon the strict, decisive, unequivocal exactitude that separates ordinary conversation from what goes on in court. Most people outside the legal profession find the verbiage daunting, its questions indecipherable, its procedures confusing and its forensic literality overwhelming. But for someone who is already multiply disadvantaged to enter the legal corridors of power, of linguistic parlance, of attention to the tiniest flaw or careless trip in an attempt to prove innocence, it can be an impossible task. Not only does legal process have its own professional vocabulary or jargon, but the very business of its system is evidence-based and language-based, focusing on the nuances of expression, coherence, accuracy and fact. In this context it is not surprising that those people who have slipped the detection they required most – that is the detection of their specific learning difficulty in childhood – can find themselves rejected by every system – home, school, workplace – and then finally when they find themselves inveigled into crime they do not have the capacity to tell their story in a way that does not disadvantage them further.

Before I proceed any further it is very important to stress that only a small minority of people with a specific learning difficulty find themselves in such extreme circumstances as to be in trouble with the law; most, like me, just get on with it and deal with the cards they were dealt. However, children in the educational system with undetected or untreated specific learning difficulties ultimately cause an unnecessary and costly burden on government departments, namely Education and Health, and the judiciary services. When children with difficulties receive either inappropriate or no intervention, some can, understandably, go on to develop associated negative emotional and behavioural problems. As time goes by and they feel more and more excluded and less and less understood, they often become less receptive and less compliant at school and also less amenable to intervention if it is too little and too late. Many either slip through the education system unnoticed and become the under-achievers, or they can fall out of the system altogether to become the early school leavers. This is a tragedy because their difficulties could have been remediated during the school years if only they had been recognised and a standard appropriate individual assessment carried out with specific follow-up intervention.

Of course children who do not receive the help they need may develop associated problems. It is not surprising that some become disillusioned, disruptive, truant or even delinquent in an effort to have some sense of power and control somewhere in their lives, if only the power of a can of paint to graffiti a wall with the tragic irony of misspelt outrage against society and how it has neglected them. That scenario can lead to more serious consequences over time, as these children grow into adults.

In July 1999, Britain's Channel 4 screened a very powerful series called 'Dyslexia Season', which examined the research available at that time on dyslexia, which estimated that there were 375,000 children in Britain with dyslexia. The series included a documentary study called *Dyslexic Criminals* which was conducted by Dr Gavin Reid, a psychologist and senior lecturer in the Faculty of Education at Edinburgh University, and Jane Kirk, the university's dyslexia study adviser. The study was based in Polmont Young Offenders Institute near Edinburgh and it explored the possible link between undetected dyslexia and crime. The study tested the theory that undiagnosed dyslexia and criminality are inextricably linked. A random sample of fifty inmates with a variety of convictions – including burglary, car theft, drug offences and assault – had volunteered to take part and all were assessed for dyslexia. Surprisingly, 25 of the volunteer sample of 50 were diagnosed as having dyslexia; that's an amazing 50 per cent. Furthermore, from the total number of 300 Polmont young offenders:

- 82 per cent had been school truants.
- 83 per cent had been suspended from school on at least one occasion.
- Over 50 per cent had been expelled from school.

The Channel 4 documentary also reported findings from a Metropolitan Police study of crimes in the Greater London area around the same time stating that 50 per cent of all burglaries and 40 per cent of all muggings were perpetrated by truanting schoolchildren.

Coincidentally, in the same year a longitudinal study was published,[12] which revealed that 25 per cent of pupils followed in the Mannheim prospective longitudinal study who were diagnosed as dyslexic at eight years of age had criminal proceedings against them by eighteen years of age. These are all alarming statistics, which haven't changed over time.

Thankfully, there is more and more awareness that a large percentage of adolescents and adults who are detained within the juvenile justice services or the adult prison services have, to some degree, language and literacy difficulties which have largely gone undetected or untreated. In 2012 the Dyslexia Foundation in Britain reported that:

- 80 per cent of all school truants were dyslexic.
- 70 per cent of young offenders were dyslexic.
- 50 per cent of the prison population was dyslexic.

These findings concur with previous studies and are shocking statistics in this modern era. In the Irish context, in 2003 the results of a survey commissioned by the Department of Justice, Equality and Law Reform[13] revealed that a significant number of prisoners were functionally illiterate, with 52 per cent of them at a pre-literacy stage in that they could identify the alphabet and write their names but were otherwise unable to read or write.

So what are the implications of someone with a specific learning difficulty becoming involved in the legal system and, in particular, the criminal justice process? The correlation between criminal conduct and difficulties with literacy skills at different stages of the criminal justice process does deserve serious research attention. We know only too well the connection between criminal conduct and experiences of social isolation and the frustration of not being able to engage in society because of difficulties with reading and writing at the most basic levels. One of the stages when those with literacy problems have evident difficulty is during the process for applying for bail before the District Court. If an accused person is refused bail before this court an application can then be made to the High Court. In previous times, the High Court bail list was divided into two lists. List A was for applicants who were represented by a solicitor. List B was for those who filed their own application papers and were not legally represented. A recurring and frequent characteristic of the applications that comprised List B was that the applicants did not actually fill out their own form, because they simply did not have the requisite literacy skills to do so. It is understood that a significant quantity of the applications for List B were completed through the assistance of persons employed by the Irish Prison Service.

In more recent times, there is now only one bail list and the established practice became that of solicitors swearing affidavits on behalf of their clients. However, this practice too has now been terminated and applicants for bail now have to swear their own affidavits. It remains to be seen if this will make manifest again the patent difficulties which many people who are brought before the Irish courts for serious criminal conduct have with basic literacy skills.

So, looking at the implications in more detail, reading and spelling skills are on the oral–literate continuum, which is simply a way of thinking about the stages of language development that starts with oral language skills (what you can say and understand in conversation) and advances towards literacy skills that would be regarded as a more advanced level of language representation because they involve reading and writing the language. With this in mind, all the skills linked to language development and subsequent literacy development have to be considered.

In the context of legal or criminal proceedings, having a difficulty in any of these areas can have a negative impact on how a person behaves and this can lead to misunderstandings or even a misrepresentation of the motives of the alleged offender. I wouldn't for one minute condone or excuse criminal behaviour, but I do believe that in some cases, when someone finds themselves in trouble with the law, the bigger picture might need closer scrutiny.

Firstly, regarding oral language development, when a person reaches adolescence or adulthood they are expected to have developed competent language skills, but for many this is just not the case. Language development is a very complex area and I will try to simplify it again by looking at four main areas:

- Receptive language skills, otherwise known as the understanding or comprehension of language that is heard
- Expressive language skills, which is the ability to express yourself easily; in other words to be able to say what you want to say and get your message across when talking
- Speech, which encompasses expressing ideas and thoughts clearly and fluently in words and sentences; it also involves speech clarity and correct pronunciation of sounds and words
- Pragmatics, or the social use of language: dealing with eye contact, following a flow of thought, being able to listen, not interrupting or dominating a conversation but turn-taking in conversation, understanding the nuances of language or

situations, showing emotions that are right for the occasion, and so on

If an adolescent or adult finds it hard to understand what is being said – or in other words has poor receptive language skills – their knowledge and understanding of words, or vocabulary, tends to be depressed. This is a very common pattern with poor or reluctant readers. This generally means that they get confused when they are spoken to in advanced, elaborate language, or when complex vocabulary or embedded sentences (which are small statements or comments placed within a sentence to give more information, e.g. 'my colleague, who is very unwell, cannot attend the meeting') are used. On top of that, they may have to deal with legal or technical jargon or wording which, to be fair, can be a mystery to most of us. As a result, they might misinterpret or simply not understand formal questions that are being put to them by a police officer, solicitor, barrister or judge. As mentioned previously, people who have significant language or literacy difficulties also tend to have poor listening skills, short attention spans or weak short-term working memory, which can cause a whole range of difficulties, such as:

- They are unable to stay focused on the questions being asked because their mind wanders to associated thoughts or worries.
- They quickly reach a language or processing overload; it gets too much having to listen, concentrate and answer, so they just switch off.
- They quickly forget the information being given to them so they don't know how to respond and can't formulate a logical response.

- They might misinterpret part or all of a question, which results in them responding either inappropriately or not at all.
- They might need a longer time to process or understand a question or information or the implications of what is being said. This can irk the person waiting for an answer and could be misinterpreted as defiance or noncompliance.
- Inappropriate and possibly unintentional responses can worsen a situation and lead to the possibility of further disciplinary actions – getting it wrong, saying the wrong thing, contradicting what they said and getting so tied up in knots that they seem guilty anyway.
- They can be easily distracted by extraneous sounds, noise, nearby conversations and activity around them. This is very common for people who have auditory processing sensitivity or central auditory processing disorders.
- They may need to move, rock or fidget a lot, which is subconsciously done to aid memory, focus and comprehension. This reflects an underlying sensory integration difficulty, but if misunderstood can again lead to the listener becoming irritated and thus further repercussions.
- They may try to camouflage their lack of understanding by looking defiant or disinterested.

If an adolescent or adult has poor expressive language skills, their use of vocabulary will be limited and will often present as immature. Additional problems can then arise:

- Many will have 'word-finding' difficulties, particularly when they are under pressure or stressed, often overusing terms like 'yoke' or 'thing'.
- Many will have difficulty remembering people's names or place names when under pressure.

- Depending on the jargon in their social group, they may use vernacular words or urban lingo, which can be as confusing to the listener as the legalese used by their legal representatives is to them.
- Many will be unable to get their point of view across in a clear and succinct way and this stumbling and stalling might be misinterpreted as guilt or lack of a credible story rather than lack of linguistic skill.
- As sequencing (that is the order of events: what comes first, second, third, etc.) is usually an issue, many have trouble getting a sequence of events in the correct order, which can give the impression that they are making parts up and telling an unlikely tale when they are just telling their story incoherently.
- Directionality and left–right orientation is often an issue, so describing scenes or giving directions can be problematic, which again can give the impression of being vague or elusive.
- If they can't express themselves clearly some will stay silent, again possibly appearing to be uncooperative, oppositional or evasive.

When an adolescent or adult has poor articulation or speech production, they will avoid speaking publicly for fear of ridicule. Large multisyllabic words can be jumbled or might have internal syllables omitted (e.g. 'vincinity' for 'vicinity' or 'accommdation' for 'accommodation'), particularly if there is a marked literacy problem evident. Those with fluency disorders like stammering (which is getting stuck on certain words or sounds, e.g. 'mmmm-man') might also avoid speaking in unfamiliar settings or to people they don't know, for fear that the stress will make their stammer worse. Articulation and fluency disorders are not uncommon with language or specific learning difficulties and can often be the first obvious sign that there is an underlying problem.

Adolescents and adults with poor pragmatic language or social skills can sometimes find themselves in trouble without really knowing or understanding how they got there in the first place. People with pragmatic language skills have some of the following difficulties:

- They can be unable to establish or maintain eye contact.
- They may misread situations and react inappropriately.
- They may not pick up the nuances of language and might take humour or sarcasm literally, thus causing or receiving offence when none was intended.
- They can interpret language or instructions literally, which can cause problems.
- They may not understand idioms, i.e. phrases such as 'throwing in the towel'.
- They tend to get into trouble easily.
- They often become the scapegoat.
- They feel or become awkward in certain situations, which again can be misinterpreted as guilt or defiance.
- They can be poor at interpreting or comprehending unspoken rules, which leads them into trouble.
- They can misinterpret body language, which again can get them into trouble.
- They may respond to dares without considering the full implications of their actions.

Any of these issues could contribute towards and sometimes compound a situation for an offender when they are involved in the criminal justice system. Having any of these difficulties is bad enough, but it becomes even more complicated when reading and spelling difficulties are also added into the mix, which might be separate to or in association with any language deficit.

Let's now look at the other end of the oral–literate continuum, namely that of literacy. As we already know, a large percentage of inmates within the prison population have specific learning difficulties. So how does it affect their situation? As explained previously, people with low-level literacy skills don't normally achieve academically, which affects them into adulthood. This makes it difficult for them to secure skilled employment and they often end up in unskilled lower-paid jobs or unemployed. They can be faced with multiple challenges and some resort to criminal activities to supplement their income. Just like the language component, literacy is also a very complex area that I will address in three broad areas:

- Reading
- Spelling
- Written expression

To read competently you need to be able to do three things. Firstly, you need to be able to decode or break down written words. Secondly, you need to be able to understand what you have just read. Thirdly, you need to be able to read at a sufficient speed that allows for comprehension; reading either too quickly or too slowly distorts comprehension. From a personal perspective, at this stage of my own dyslexic journey I am now 'consciously competent' at reading; in other words, when faced with an unfamiliar word I can apply my own strategies to work the word out, so I am rarely thrown. However, reading comprehension remains a challenge for me and one I frequently encounter when filling out forms or reading legal or official documents. So I now have a good level of literacy and can deal with most things that I come across. But I can still remember the earlier times and I know how unsettling it is to fill in forms, for example, when you have reading difficulties. For anyone with an ongoing literacy problem some of the possible implications that can arise include:

- They may have an inability to deal with official letters or documents, by either ignoring them or putting them on the long finger and missing deadlines. The filling out of forms and the implications of not doing so became very obvious to me recently while I filled out the 2016 Census form, which is a legal obligation. Without a doubt, a competent level of literacy is required to both read and complete this form. Failure to do so can lead to a fine of up to a staggering €45,500. It would be most interesting to know how many of these forms were not filled out due to low levels of literacy and, if this is the case, what the repercussions, if any, actually were.
- They may not read important notices, e.g. understand a solicitor's written advice.
- They may not check their own important submissions, e.g. personal details or statements, to ensure the information is accurate.
- They may misread written documents, e.g. appointments, instructions or requests, resulting in problems of non-compliance.
- They may not be able to read or understand maps or timetables.
- They may feel frustrated or embarrassed at being totally reliant on others, e.g. to show them what to do or tell them where to be.

A difficulty with spelling is not as problematic nowadays with modern technology providing predictive text, spell checking and access to dictionaries. In addition, many more people are poor spellers than poor readers and it seems to be more acceptable across all levels of society to own up to being a poor speller. Nonetheless, if the difficulty is severe, dyslexic people may not be able to complete mandatory forms or respond to written communications as indicated within the documents.

When someone has a difficulty with oral expression it will normally, but not always, be reflected in their written expression. Some people need time to write something, which allows them to formulate their thoughts, because when there is time pressure to write a submission then difficulties with content, thought sequencing, layout or penmanship may be apparent. This can alert a parent, teacher or other professional that there could be underlying language or literacy problems that should be followed up. This problem really struck me when I attended a Restorative Justice Conference in May 2016. While attending one presentation in particular, the presenter described how restorative practices can be utilised within a custodial setting as part of the process of community reintegration. She described a project she was engaged in which involved working with adult offenders and their victims in Ireland. One of the restorative justice interventions employed was for the offender to write an apology letter to their victim, which reflected their understanding of the cause and effect of their actions. In participating in this project it is understood that the offender was then given a more lenient sentence from the presiding judge in their case. While this is a very commendable practice and one to be promoted, what if the offender can't either formulate their thoughts in a meaningful way or express them coherently in writing? Are they then disadvantaged from a sentencing perspective as well?

Of course, having any of these problems can have a negative impact on the emotional well-being or mental health of the individual concerned. The occurrence of stress and anxiety-related disorders, low self-esteem and low self-confidence can result in their coping mechanisms being undermined or compromised. They can become angry or seem to be incompetent in certain situations, and in order to gain acceptance they might be easily influenced or easily led. The longer these behaviours continue, the more difficult it is to change them.

For many offenders and inmates, the shame attached to having a specific language impairment or specific learning difficulty is stronger than that of serving time as the punishment for their crime. Adolescents and adults within these services who demonstrate a vulnerability in this area should be offered a speech and language assessment. Thankfully, speech and language therapists are now beginning to be employed within the young offender and prison services, so there may be some light at the end of the tunnel. I strongly believe that all governments have a responsibility to rehabilitate inmates and offenders back into society. By offering those who need it the opportunity for a language and literacy assessment with follow-up intervention, we can give them a better opportunity in life, and a sense of hope, which might stop them returning to a cycle of crime and reoffending.

***

This chapter explores the extreme situations that a small minority of people with an undiagnosed or untreated specific learning difficulty may find themselves in with the law. It points out signs to be alert to when dealing with this population so that genuine cases are not misunderstood.

Support to Access the World of Written Words

If there is one idea that has dominated this book it is that we live in a literate world where everyone has, or should have, the right to an education. Fundamentally, literacy is the cornerstone of our education process because if you don't learn to read then you can't read to learn. Regardless of what technologies we develop, not requiring the written word and the capacity to read it is unimaginable. Despite voice-activated technology with which to 'write' what we wish to say and audio technology to 'read' for us what we need to hear, literacy still rules and is a human access right and entitlement.

Of course, educationally everything is changing and digital technology is rapidly altering the way we learn by giving us fingertip access to masses of information. This makes our reading, processing and curating skills all the more important. But with the rapidity of the changes in technology, teaching practices are in a state of flux, endlessly adapting to the rate and pace of change. Nothing is fixed. Nothing is static. We are in a new educational era in terms of how information comes to us and how we communicate what we know to others. For those parents and teachers who remember a time when technology played a lesser part in the core of educational practices there is the constant challenge of keeping up with new and evolving communication platforms and content. Teachers and parents are always engaged in trying to understand the manner and extent to which technology shapes the interests and ambitions of the younger generation, most of whom are more digitally savvy than the previous generation. And let us not forget that a 'generation' in terms of technology or digital design can be as short as two to three years. The neuronal wiring of those babies who hold an iPad as quickly as they hold a toy is a wonder to behold.

I was recently sitting on a bus beside a young mother with her son. I noticed the child had a very limited vocabulary and I thought that he was probably aged somewhere between eighteen months and two years of age. The little boy was becoming restless and his mother gave him her phone to quieten him down. It was fascinating to watch the child manipulate his mother's phone to play, replay and interact with what turned out to be a *Peppa Pig* app. It brought home to me just how technically confident toddlers are nowadays. We, the older generations, are sometimes referred to as 'dinosaurs', and I think this is mainly because quite a few of us are afraid of change and technology. Of course there are always generation gaps between each generation, but to reach young people, to speak their language and be active participants in their technological world, we need to become at least digitally aware. Thankfully, technology is becoming increasingly user-friendly for all ages.

Technology: love it or loath it, you can't get away from it. A report on the BBC Breakfast News recently suggested that students from the ages of seven to thirteen spend, on average, three hours a day on their computers or electronic devices. The probability is that most of this time is being spent on social media instagramming, snapchatting, tweeting and gaming. The good news is that this technology, which the kids find enjoyable, is being used for learning activities too. Be it a smartphone, tablet, laptop or computer, the fact is that the educational programmes available on these devices can and do stimulate interaction and engagement. This not only applies to the regular learning population but also to people with learning and/or other disabilities. By and large there are a huge number of free or inexpensive apps for education that are available online 24 hours a day. Amongst the great examples of technology benefiting all of us are the massive open online courses (MOOCs) from many universities providing unlimited participation and open access via the web. They can certainly make a real difference in levelling the playing field, especially for those who would not otherwise have the means to access this education and for those who are motivated to learn.

Information and communication technology (ICT) and assistive technology is so important for dyslexic students because it can alleviate the pressure of having to read, write or spell accurately. This is because most people with a specific learning difficulty have a preference for learning through the visual modality; in other words, they learn better from what they see, rather than what they hear. There are a number of advantages to using technology for those who learn differently:

- Technology is interactive; it enables the student to be hands-on and to actively engage with the learning activity. They can take control of how the information is presented, such as the speed of delivery, and they also have the opportunity to repeat what was presented as often as they like. They can work in their own time, at their own pace and in their preferred environment.
- Technology provides a multisensory approach; it is auditory, visual and manually tactile.
- Text can be spaced to fit personal preferences; diagrams, mind maps, charts, illustrations and pictograms can be

modified to eradicate visual stress. Audio volume can be adjusted to suit the listener and earphones can be worn to cut out extraneous distractions. Screen background and foreground colours and brightness can be changed, as can font size, font type and spacing to again eradicate visual strain.

- Specific apps for note-taking, text-to-speech or speech-to-text dictation, and recording facilities are essential study aids for dyslexic students. Using tools such as read-back software, text highlighters, spell checker and predictive text can all provide compensatory strategies for those with poor literacy skills.

- Audio books, which can easily be downloaded from the internet or obtained from local libraries, are excellent study tools for reluctant readers. Using such facilities means that younger students have access to books and literature that are well beyond their reading ability level. Listening to audio books will improve their overall language skills. Older students can also gain, e.g. prior to tackling a project they could listen to an audio book and/or watch the film of a play or novel on their curriculum. Other devices on the market, such as tablet computers, are also excellent in this regard as they too can be modified to individual needs. These devices also provide quick access to dictionaries, which helps the student's comprehension when they come across an unfamiliar word.

- Dyslexic students need to be organised to function properly and technology can really assist here with daily, personal, study- and work-related tasks. Using an electronic organiser or an app for a smartphone or tablet will help students to keep track of dates, schedules and deadlines, as well as recording important notes and references.

- Mind-mapping software is also excellent for organising and planning for:
  - Improving sequential thought and maintaining topic cohesion for both oral and written expression
  - Improving reading comprehension, in that students learn to recognise the important points in a text and to ignore 'padding'
  - Developing excellent factual study notes
- Other features like 'cut and paste', spell checker and grammar checker also help to make written tasks that bit easier.

The huge importance of technology as a navigation tool for severely dyslexic students came home to me with a bang recently when I reassessed an eleven-year-old boy whom I have known for a few years. As this child lived quite a distance away I only saw him sporadically but he had huge support from his wonderful parents, his teacher and local services. This child had access to and fully availed of all that was on offer. However, he is the most profoundly dyslexic child I ever worked with and no matter what was done he could not get past a preliminary stage of erratic sound–symbol association and basic high-frequency or common word recognition. The written letter, never mind word, made very little sense to him and he just could not retain what he was being taught over time. However, he loved machinery, woodwork and construction, so he took to technology like a duck to water. Whereas it had become apparent that formal literacy instruction was going to fail him no matter how hard he tried, technology with all its advancements in the area of dyslexia was going to save him and give him access at last to the world of written language and the school curriculum. With the use of technology and the availability of curriculum-based ebooks he can now access the school curriculum equally, albeit differently, to his peers.

Useful Technologies

Below we discuss some of the better current products, tools and services that are available for people with specific learning difficulties. There are so many companies providing educational products and services to schools (business to business) and to the general public (business to consumer), but there is very little advice available as to their effectiveness, other than anecdotal evidence and sales patter. Although I keep a professional eye on new developments online and through professional correspondence, events and publications, I also like to be 'hands on' and meet face-to-face with the product developers and salespeople, which is the reason I attend the British Educational Training and Technology (BETT) show in London every year. It claims to be the world's leading education technology event. Basically it's a trade show that showcases the use of the latest information technology in education. Although my main focus is always on exploring any new technology in the specific learning difficulty domain, I'm also interested in the explosion of other online materials that are now available, particularly if they really do help students to learn to read and spell. There are many online programmes or devices available that have different functionalities specifically designed for those with a specific learning difficulty. The following are examples of what I have found to be the most current and useful in practice that facilitate interventions and treatments for dyslexia, some of which were showcased at the most recent BETT show. However, do keep in mind the rapid rate at which online materials are evolving and what may be recommended today may or may not be overtaken in time.

- *WordsWorthLearning Programme*: There is no magic bullet; this is an online programme (www.wordsworthlearning.com) that teaches students how to significantly improve their reading and spelling over a relatively short time frame. Of course, this is my own programme and I am very keen to promote it because, over the last 25 years, it has produced results-based evidence for thousands of students to prove that it works. It has now been online for five years and I have researched the competition both online and at BETT and have found no other online programme that provides this affordable and available unique process and content, or the proof of efficacy that this programme provides.

- *Reader.Pen* and *Exam.Reader*: Note, the latter is currently not sanctioned for use in state exams in Ireland, but the former can be sourced at www.scanningpens.co.uk. They use simple technology and are reader pens that scan and read the text aloud. They can also highlight and define individual words and sentences.
- *The Google Dictionary* app appears to have taken over from the Franklin Speller and is regarded as one of the best dictionary/spelling apps for using on students' portable devices.
- *Assistive technology*, such as mind-mapping programmes, is designed to aid study and organisational skills. There are a variety of online mind-mapping programmes available at www.mindmapping.com and www.imindmap.com. Other popular mind-mapping programmes, such as Inspiration and Kidspiration, are available from www.jacksontechnology. com, www.urability.com or www.dyslexic.com. Check out www.bdatech.org/what-technology/mindmaps/ for further guidance on which materials best suit the individual student's needs.
- *BBC Type to Learn* and *BBC Dance Mat Typing for Kids* (6 to 11 years) are programmes for improving typing or keyboard skills, which are both available from www.bbc.co.uk/guides/ z3c6tfr. Another programme is *English Type*, which can be purchased from www.englishtype.com. All of these products

appear to be excellent teaching resources for learning typing skills.

- There are some highly recommended computer programs that help to improve comprehension by reading text aloud, providing text and picture dictionaries, helping construct sentences, and providing word predictions and spell checks. These include:
  - ◦ *TextHelp Read&Write* – software for students who struggle to read and write. This program reads out loud what you type, reads aloud a document as it is scanned, can convert audio files to text files to be saved on CD/USB, and has an advanced spell checker and word predictor. For more information check out www.texthelp.com/en-gb. This product is also available in Ireland through www.jacksontechnology.com.
  - ◦ *ClaroRead* (similar to TextHelp and Kurzweil 3000) has a facility for text to be read aloud using a wide choice of voices, and provides highlighting, audio note-taking, spelling and predictive text features. Claro has also introduced a number of new and inexpensive apps, the two most useful of which are *ClaroSpeak Plus*, which is a text-to-speech reader, and *Claro ScanPen*, which allows students to take a photo of a printed text document and, using either a finger or stylus, to point to the text, which is then read back to them. For further information visit www.clarosoftware.com and www.claro-apps.com.
  - ◦ *Kurzweil 3000* and *Kurzweil 3000-firefly* (similar to TextHelp and ClaroRead) both contain reading and writing software for students with specific learning difficulties. Some of the most useful features are: (i) it reads aloud content that is scanned, (ii) it has a highlighter facility, (iii) it organises the layout of important information taken from a document in the note-taking style that suits the

learner, e.g. mind maps or columns, (iv) it has an inbuilt spell checker, word predictor and dictionary, and (v) it can translate content into a number of languages, e.g. English, French, German and Dutch. A Spanish version is currently under development. Although Kurzweil 3000 probably provides the most functionality, it is by far the most expensive program on the market; however grants are available for eligible students. For further information visit www.kurzweilEdu.com. This product is also available in Ireland through www.jacksontechnology.com.

○ *Livescribe* offers a combination package consisting of an electronic pen with built-in audio recorder, digitalised paper and an app. You pair the pen with your smartphone or tablet using Bluetooth technology so that when you write on the paper the app will create a digital version of your note-pages on your tablet or phone. You can then convert your handwritten notes to editable, typed text. The app supports the Japanese, Chinese, English, German, Spanish, French and Italian languages. You can find out more at www.livescribe.com.

○ *Notability* is another note-taking app for smartphones and tablets to help students create study notes. It can integrate handwriting, typing, drawings, audio files and pictures that can then be accessed in the cloud with iCloud, Google Drive, AirDrop, email and Dropbox. You can find out more at www.gingerlabs.com.

○ *Speak it!* translates words typed into the app into an audio voice so you can hear the word spoken aloud. You can also cut and paste Word documents, emails and messages that will allow you to listen to the content. This app allows students to listen to text spoken aloud so they can get the information in a way that works for them. The app also highlights words as they are read and can save the spoken words as an audio file. It is available through iTunes or the Google Chrome Web Store.

○ *Dragon Naturally Speaking* is a popular voice recognition program. When you talk at normal speed your words appear on the screen almost instantly. It turns spoken words into text and executes voice commands much faster than they can be typed. Students can edit documents, send emails, search the web and use social media easily with this program. You can personalise the voice and the software can recognise and register words and phrases that you use regularly. It provides quick feedback on what you have said, so you can check the content immediately. For further information visit www.Nuance. co.uk. This product is also available in Ireland through www.jacksontechnology.com.

○ *Clicker 7* is a reading and writing software tool that allows younger children to type words and sentences which are automatically read back to them in a friendly, age-appropriate voice that is designed to appeal to children. It also provides word predictions to help with vocabulary enrichment and spelling skills. It has a built-in planning tool called 'Clicker Board' to help students prepare for writing by brainstorming, allowing them to manipulate and link words, pictures and sounds on their board. It also offers 'Voice Notes' to capture ideas prior to writing and has a 'Word Pool' facility to expand vocabulary repertoire for writing. For further information visit www.cricksoft. com/clicker.

○ *WriteOnline* is an app (and desktop) tool that provides software for older students who struggle with written expression. It provides the opportunity for students to hear back what they have written, so students can review their work to find and correct any errors. It offers the students a range of tools that support writing across the curriculum, e.g. word predictors, and vocabulary and spell checkers, all of which can help to suggest words based on the context of the writing, helping students to use more interesting words. It also includes a mind-mapping tool for brainstorming ideas. For further information visit www.cricksoft.com/writeonline.

- *Publishing companies* such as Gill Education (www.gilleducation.ie), CJ Fallon (www.cjfallon.ie) and Folens (www.folens.ie) have all supplied schools with printed matter through the decades and still continue to do so. They are all also adapting to include digital technologies to facilitate classroom learning, and are now offering digital copies of textbooks and other associated products via their websites.

Useful Agencies and Services

- Dyslexia Association of Ireland: www.dyslexia.ie. This website has a lot of useful information and also offers a range of specialist tuition services for children with dyslexia.
- Dyspraxia Association of Ireland: www.dyspraxia.ie
- HADD Ireland for people affected by ADHD: www.hadd.ie
- Association for Higher Education Access and Disability: www.ahead.ie
- British Dyslexia Association: www.bdadyslexia.org.uk. This website provides excellent articles reviewing the technology and digital materials available for students with specific learning difficulties.
- National Adult Literacy Agency: www.nala.ie
- Adult Dyslexia Organisation: www.adult-dyslexia.org
- Dyslexia Action: www.dyslexiaaction.org.uk
- Irish Association of Speech and Language Therapists: www.iaslt.ie

- Independent Speech-Language Therapists of Ireland: www.isti.ie
- Royal College of Speech and Language Therapists: www.rcslt.org
- National Educational Psychological Services (NEPS) www.education.ie/en/Schools-Colleges/Services/National-Educational-Psychological-Service-NEPS-/NEPS-Home-Page.html
- Psychological Society of Ireland: www.psihq.ie
- Association of Occupational Therapists of Ireland: www.aoti.ie
- Association of Optometrists Ireland: www.optometrists.ie

Facilities and Grants

The Department of Education and Skills (www.education.ie) provides accommodations, facilities and grants for students with a specific learning difficulty. These provisions are now widened in their scope; the criteria for eligibility has broadened and as such no longer goes under the heading of a 'specific learning difficulty', but is now re-classed as a 'learning difficulty'. The following circulars and eligibility criteria can be found on their website in the 'circulars and forms' section:

- Reasonable Accommodations at the Certificate Examinations: Instructions for Schools (RACE), which will now be amended and reissued each year, include applications for the following:
  - Provision of a reader
  - Permission to record exam answers on a tape recorder or word processor
  - Use of a scribe
  - Waiver from the assessment of spelling, grammar and punctuation in language subjects
  - The provision of extra time (10 minutes per hour or part thereof), which is only provided to those for whom the

use of a scribe has been sanctioned, or to those who need to use a recording device or word processor, or for candidates with visual impairment

○ Sanction to take the exam in a separate room

- Circulars related to applications for an exemption from the study of Irish:
  ○ Primary school: Circular 12/96
  ○ Secondary school: Circular M10/94 (Note: There is no circular available for applying for an exemption from the study of a modern language; however different colleges, where applicable, have their own individual exemption criteria. Please check with the course/college in question to ascertain eligibility.)
- Circular 0010/2013, which relates to the scheme of grants for the purchase of essential assistive technology equipment for students

***

While the resources, facilities and grants described in this chapter are available at time of writing, many more will come on stream, some of them will be altered and adapted, and Department of Education provisions, criteria and facilities may change over time. What will not change is children's need to have their individual learning styles, differences or difficulties identified and accommodated so that they do not suffer the pain of feeling different when what they need is simply to learn differently.

Remember, if you have even the slightest notion that something isn't quite as it should be with your child's literacy development, DO SOMETHING ABOUT IT. It's never too late and you will almost certainly give your child a better opportunity to reach their true academic and life potential.

Endnotes

Chapter 1

[1] *Report of the Task Force on Dyslexia* (2001, p. xii).
[2] O'Regan, E. (2014).

Chapter 2

[3] Sheridan (1997).

Chapter 3

[4] Elliot and Grigorenko (2014, pp. 152–160).
[5] Hyatt, Stephenson and Carter (2009).
[6] Plourde et al. (2015); Snowling and Hulme (2012).

Chapter 4

[7] Elliott and Grigorenko (2014, p. 25), citing Bishop and Snowling (2004).
[8] American Psychiatric Association (2013).

Chapter 6

[9] Sandman-Hurley (2013).

Chapter 7

[10] Pinantoan (2013).
[11] Eivers and Creaven (2013, pp. 123–125).

Chapter 9

[12] Warnke (1999).

[13] Morgan and Kett (2003).

REFERENCES

American Psychiatric Association (2013) *Diagnostic and Statistical Manual of Mental Disorders*, fifth edition (DSM-5), Arlington, VA: American Psychiatric Publishing.

Bishop, D.V.M. and Snowling, M.J. (2004) 'Developmental Dyslexia and Specific Language Impairment: Same or Different?', *Psychological Bulletin*, 130(6): 858–886.

Eivers, E. and Creaven, A.M. (2013) 'Home–School Interaction' in E. Eivers and A. Clerkin (eds), *National Schools, International Contexts: Beyond the PIRIS and TIMSS Test Results*, pp. 105–128, Dublin: Educational Research Centre.

Elliot, J. and Grigorenko, E. (2014) *The Dyslexia Debate*, New York, NY: Cambridge University Press.

Hyatt, K., Stephenson, J. and Carter, M. (2009) 'A Review of Three Controversial Educational Practices: Perceptual Motor Programs, Sensory Integration, and Tinted Lenses', *Education and Treatment of Children*, 32(2): 313–342.

Morgan, M. and Kett, M. (2003) *The Prison Adult Literacy Survey: Results and Implications*, Dublin: Irish Prison Service.

O'Regan, E. (2014) 'Effects of Mild Lack of Oxygen at Birth "Long-Term"', *Irish Independent*, Health & Living Supplement, 13 January.

Pinantoan, A. (2013) 'The Effect of Parental Involvement in School and Education [Infographic]', *informED*, www.opencolleges.edu.au/informed/features/the-effect-of-parental-involvement-in-academic-achievement, 25 June.

Plourde, V., Boivin, M., Forget-Dubois, N., Brendgen, M., Vitaro, F., Marino, C., Tremblay, R. and Dionne, G. (2015) 'Phenotypic and Genetic Associations between Reading Comprehension, Decoding Skills, and ADHD

References

Dimensions: Evidence from Two Population-Based Studies', *Journal of Child Psychology and Psychiatry*, 56(10): 1074–1082.

Sandman-Hurley, K. (2013) 'What Is Dyslexia?', TED-Ed, http://ed.ted.com/lessons/what-is-dyslexia-kelli-sandman-hurley.

Sheridan, M. (1997) *From Birth to Five Years: Children's Developmental Progress*, London: Routledge.

Snowling, M. and Hulme, C. (2012) 'Annual Research Review: The Nature and Classification of Reading Disorders – A Commentary on Proposals for DSM-5', *Journal of Child Psychology and Psychiatry*, 53(5): 593–607.

Task Force on Dyslexia (2001) *Report of the Task Force on Dyslexia*, Special Education Support Service, Department of Education and Skills, http://www.sess.ie/sites/default/files/Dyslexia_Task_Force_Report_0.pdf.

Warnke, A. (1999) 'Reading and Spelling Disorders: Clinical Features and Causes', *European Child & Adolescent Psychiatry* 8(Suppl. 3): S2–S12.

Glossary

Adenoids: lymphatic tissue situated between the back of the nose and the throat

Anoxia: an absence or deficiency of oxygen reaching the brain and organs of the body

Articulation: speech production using the tongue, teeth, lips and palate

Asperger's syndrome: also known as high-functioning autism, is characterised by diminished ability with social communication and interaction

Assessments: standardised tests to evaluate an individual's performance on certain tasks compared to their peer group, e.g. for reading or spelling

Assistive technology: any device or program, such as a laptop or voice recognition software, which assists the individual in communicating, absorbing or producing information

Attainment tests: standardised tests for reading accuracy, reading comprehension, spelling or mathematics

Attention: an individual's ability to listen, focus and concentrate on auditory or visual information

Attention deficit (hyperactivity) disorder (ADHD): a genetic condition that affects an individual's attention span, learning and behaviour right through childhood and in many cases beyond into adulthood

Audiologist: a professional who assesses an individual's hearing acuity or ability

Auditory memory: the ability to remember what is heard

Auditory processing: an individual's ability to hear, recognise, process, order and remember speech sounds in a word or words in a sentence

Autistic spectrum disorders (ASDs): neurological disorders that affect both children and adults, characterised by difficulties with social communication and interaction, and with social imagination and flexible thinking

Behavioural optometrist: a professional who checks if an individual has a reduced ability to make sense of what they see, despite having normal vision

Biological: related to biology or life patterns or behaviours

CAMHS: Child and adolescent mental health service

Case history: a record of an individual's personal history, often used to assist with their diagnosis and treatment

Central auditory processing disorders (CAPD): when an individual is struggling to understand what they hear, despite having normal hearing

Chronological age: an individual's actual age

Clinical psychologist: a professional who focuses on diagnosing and treating mental, emotional, learning and behavioural disorders

Cognitive assessment: a formal standardised assessment of an individual's intelligence

Collaboration: when the parent, teacher/other professional and student are all involved in working together to improve the student's learning and progress

Communication: the ability to convey your message through speech, gestures, body language, facial expressions or written words

Comorbid: when two or more conditions are coexisting in the same person

Concentration: the ability to fully attend to or focus on something

Consonants: all the letters of the alphabet excluding A, E, I, O, U (the vowels); some would also regard Y as a vowel rather than a consonant letter, as it has the function of a vowel

Convergence: involves bringing the eyes together to follow something coming towards them at close proximity

DAI: Dyslexia Association of Ireland

Decoding: another term for reading, which involves the breaking down and re-blending of letters into their respective speech sounds (phonemes), rules and syllables, and assigning meaning to them

Decoding disorder: another term for a serious reading difficulty

Delay: a term used when a person is developing along the normal developmental milestones but at a slower pace than usual

Glossary

Developmental dyslexia: a reading and/or spelling disorder that is of biological or neurological origin

Developmental milestones: the ages and stages that children are expected to be able to show a skill, e.g. walking or babbling

Diagnosis: when a specialist assesses and identifies a disease or disorder in an individual

Differential diagnosis: the process of differentiating between two or more conditions which share similar signs or symptoms

Digital technology: devices that use digital code to transmit signals and information between different devices, e.g. mobile phones, computers, tablets

Disorder: a significant disturbance in the normal expected developmental patterns in an area of learning, or neurological or physical development

Drumcondra reading test: a primary school group reading test that consists of multiple-choice questions covering three categories: reading vocabulary (understanding what words mean), reading comprehension (understanding sentences or texts read silently), and word analysis (ability to recognise words with similar sound and spelling patterns). The overall reading scores are calculated on the students' combined scores on the reading vocabulary and reading comprehension subtests only.

DSM-5 (*Diagnostic and Statistical Manual*, fifth edition): the standard classification of mental disorders

Dysgraphia: a difficulty with handwriting and the ability to produce written work legibly and quickly by hand

Dyslexia: a neurodevelopmental disorder which is a continuum of specific learning difficulties related to the acquisition of basic skills in reading, spelling and/or writing, such difficulties being unexplained in relation to an individual's other abilities and educational experiences

Dyspraxia (developmental coordination disorder (DCD)): marked difficulties with movement and specific aspects of learning such as with thinking out, planning, organising and carrying out visual, motor or sensory tasks

Educational psychologist: a professional who works with children and young people to assess and support their educational, emotional and behavioural development

Encoding: another term for spelling, which involves working out the speech sounds and corresponding letters, and the rules and syllables embedded in a word when writing it

Encoding disorder: another term for a serious spelling difficulty

Evidence-based practice: the integration of clinical expertise, scientific research and client values and requirements to provide the best intervention approach for an individual

Expressive language skills: the ability to express yourself easily; in other words, to be able to say what you want to say and get your message across when talking

Familial: something related to or occurring in the family

Fine/gross motor difficulties: when an individual shows difficulty with fine motor skills (e.g. writing, opening/closing buttons or tying laces) or gross motor skills (e.g. throwing, kicking or catching a ball, hopping, skipping, jumping or riding a bike)

Flipped classroom: an educational model which involves creating and providing lessons online, outside of the classroom, which allows the student to view the lesson content in their own time, at their own pace and in their preferred environment; these lessons are then reinforced back in the classroom setting

Fluency: the ability to speak easily and not, for example, stumble or stutter over words

Full scale IQ score: a term used to describe an individual's complete cognitive ability score across several parameters or measures on a given standardised test

Gaelscoil: an all-Irish speaking school

GAI (global ability index): a composite score that is based on three verbal comprehension and three perceptual reasoning subtests, and does not include the working memory or processing speed subtests included in the full-scale IQ measurement; this is normally used when there is a large discrepancy across the four areas measured that would result in an overall distorted IQ profile

Genetic: hereditary information held in the individual's genes or chromosomes

Grammar: established rules of a language to demonstrate the relationship between classes of words in a sentence

Grommet: a plastic tube surgically implanted in the eardrum to drain fluid from the middle ear, which can alleviate fluctuating hearing problems

HIE (hypoxic-ischaemic encephalopathy): a brain injury caused by oxygen deprivation to the brain

ICT (information and communication technology): the distribution of information across technology such as the internet

Idiom: an expression not to be taken literally, e.g. 'over the moon'

IEP (individual educational plan): an intervention programme designed to focus on an individual's profile of needs

Intellectual disability: when an individual's intelligence is scored below the average range of ability

Intervention: a therapy approach to modify or change a result for the better

IQ (intelligence quotient): a number which shows an individual's intelligence level; a score of 100 is average

Irlen lenses or overlays: tinted glasses or overlays for the treatment of scotopic sensitivity syndrome. There is controversy regarding whether or not this visual condition actually exists and it is not recognised by the medical profession, nor are the use of Irlen lenses or overlays recommended.

Jargon: technical or professional wording

Language exemption: permission given to a student by the Department of Education and Science to exclude the mandatory learning of Irish or a modern language on clearly defined medical, educational or social grounds

Learning support: additional educational support provided in schools for weaker students by specially designated learning support teachers

Letter–sound correspondence: the matching of a letter to a speech sound, e.g. 'p' sounds like /puh/

Literacy: the ability to read and write

Long vowels: for example /ae, ee, ie, oe, ue/ where you say the letter name and not the sound, e.g. /ae/ in 'bathe' as opposed to the short vowel /a/ in 'bath'

Malapropism: misuse of one word for another that sounds like it, e.g. to be 'pacific' instead of 'specific'

Mechanics of reading or spelling: knowing 'how' to read and spell

MICRA-T reading test: a group test to provide Irish primary school teachers with information on the reading levels of pupils in their classes

Mind mapping: a study tool for making visual notes of school texts and other information; it assists in the comprehension and retention of information

Mixed metaphor: when two or more common idioms are mixed together to give an illogical phrase, e.g. 'I can read him like the back of my book'

Motor development: the development of physical movement

Multidisciplinary team: professionals from different fields working together, e.g. doctors, psychologists, and speech and language therapists

NARA II (Neale Analysis of Reading Ability – second edition): a tool used by educational psychologists, teachers, and speech and language therapists to measure reading ability across three parameters: accuracy, comprehension and rate

NEPS (National Educational Psychological Service): a Department of Education and Science agency of psychologists who specialise in working in schools with the school-age population

Occupational therapist (OT): a health professional who assesses and treats different health conditions which can affect people's abilities to function normally; they help people to overcome or work around the difficulties that are affecting their daily occupations or lifestyles

Oculomotor dysfunction: a difficulty with visual tracking or 'convergence', which involves bringing the eyes closer together to follow something coming towards them at close proximity, or 'accommodation', which involves being able to switch the eye focus from long distance to short distance

Oculomotor function: eye movements

Optometrist: a specialist who examines patients' eyes and diagnoses and prescribes treatment before referring patients to medical practitioners if necessary

Oral–literate continuum: a way of thinking about some of the stages of language development; it is an extension of oral language development (how one speaks) into written language (how one writes)

Oral commands: spoken instructions

Oral language processing disorder: an impairment in the development and use of language due to difficulties in language comprehension and/or speech or language production

Orally tactile or oral kinaesthetic feedback: how to shape or place the tongue, teeth and lips to make a particular sound and the *feeling* of the sound being made

Otitis media or glue ear: a painful type of ear infection that occurs when the area behind the eardrum, called the middle ear, becomes inflamed and infected

Paired reading: when an adult and a child take turns reading aloud together

Panacea: a cure for all ills

Peers: individuals of one's own age group

Percentile ranking (PR): shows a child's position compared against 100 others of the same age. For example, a PR score of 10 would mean that 90 per cent of the population of that age group would have scored higher on that particular test. On most standardised tests the average scores range from the 25th to the 75th percentile rankings. So, if your child scores in the 25th percentile (the bottom end of average) there would be 75 in the group with a better score and 24 with a lesser score.

Phonemes: individual speech sounds; there are approximately 44 in the English language

Phonemic approach: speech–sound approach to teaching reading and spelling

Phonetics: the relationship between a letter and a sound

Phonic approach: letter–sound approach to teaching reading and spelling

Phonological processing disorder: a problem with being able to recognise the rules that govern a language in order to break down a word into separate speech sounds or phonemes and then associate each of those sounds with the letters that make up the word

Pragmatics: the social use of language, dealing with eye contact, following a flow of thought, being able to listen, not interrupting or dominating a conversation but turn-taking in conversation, understanding the nuances of language or situations, showing emotions that are right for the occasion, and so on

Pre-reading and pre-spelling stage of literacy: the earliest stage of reading and spelling development, where the student is being introduced to letters and sounds but cannot yet read or write

Glossary

Prefix: a syllable added to the beginning of a word to create a new word with a different meaning, e.g. 'un' + 'happy' = 'unhappy', 'multi' + 'cultural' = 'multicultural'

Processing sensory information: making sense of and responding to sensory information or what we see, hear, smell, touch or feel around us

Professionals: a person qualified in a profession; in this book it refers generally to general practitioners (GPs), psychiatrists, psychologists, speech and language therapists, occupational therapists, teachers, audiologists and behavioural optometrists

Prognosis: the expected outcome of a condition

Pseudo-words: nonsense/made-up words

Psychiatrist: a medical doctor who specialises in the branch of medicine devoted to the diagnosis, prevention, study, and treatment of mental health disorders

Psychological assessment: a process of testing cognitive abilities and behaviours, as well as assessing literacy and numeracy skills

Psychologist: a professional who assesses and studies the role of mental functions in individual and social behaviour; they also explore the physiological and biological processes that underlie cognitive functions and behaviours

Psychosomatic complaints: physical symptoms that occur for psychological reasons (e.g. stress) and impair an individual's ability to function normally

Reading/spelling delay: the development of reading and spelling skills along normal developmental lines but at a slower rate than would be expected for a person's age level

Reading/spelling disorder (also known as an decoding/encoding disorder): the erratic development of reading and spelling skills, which would not be along normal developmental lines and would be at a slower rate than would be expected for a person's age and ability

Reading comprehension: the ability to understand what is read

Reasonable accommodations: special arrangements made for students with permanent or long-term conditions, e.g. visual and hearing difficulties, or specific learning difficulties, which will facilitate them in taking state examinations; examples of accommodations are waivers for spelling and grammar, or the provision or a reader or scribe

Receptive language: comprehension or understanding of the spoken or written word

Remedial/remediation: provision of a remedy or cure for something

Resource teacher: a teacher who works with children who have additional educational needs, over and above those catered for by the learning support teacher in the school setting. These children must have a psychological report and a diagnosis which entitles them to a certain number of hours of additional, normally one-to-one, support.

Results-based evidence: using therapy outcomes to demonstrate the effectiveness of an intervention

Rhinitis: inflammation of the mucus membrane in the nose; children with rhinitis can often have other concomitant ear, nose and throat problems, which can adversely affect the ability to hear and then learn

Scotopic sensitivity syndrome: a physical discomfort, e.g. sore eyes or headaches, due to a glare caused by reflective light on reading materials. It is a sensitivity to light. There is controversy regarding whether or not this visual condition actually exists and it is not recognised by the medical profession.

Sensory integration difficulties: difficulties with movement and specific aspects of learning such as with thinking things through, planning, organising and carrying out motor or sensory tasks

Short vowels: these are /a, e, i, o, u/ where you say the sound and not the letter name, e.g. /a/ in 'bath' as opposed to the long vowel /ae/ in 'bathe'

Siblings: brothers or sisters

Speech and language therapist (SLT): a professional who assesses, diagnoses and treats a variety of speech, language, learning, voice, fluency and communication problems with children and adults

Social cues: the signals that individuals send through body language and facial expressions

Social function: the ability to engage appropriately in social situations; those who cannot often appear emotionally immature

Socialisation: the process of learning socially acceptable behaviours and mixing socially with others

Specific language impairment (SLI) (formally called a specific language disorder and more recently renamed as a developmental language disorder): a disordered development of receptive (comprehension) and expressive language skills

Specific learning difficulty: an unexpected difficulty with learning age-appropriate reading, spelling, writing or mathematical skills despite having normal intellectual ability. It describes the gap between a person's academic potential and actual ability.

Speech and language deficit: a disordered development of receptive (comprehension) and expressive language skills, though not as severe as an SLI

Speech: how sounds or words are spoken; also how an individual expresses ideas and thoughts clearly and fluently in words and sentences

Standard deviations (SD): a statistical method for calculating where a child's performance on a test is placed in the average band, i.e. ranging from well-below average to well-above average. 0 is the average score, -1 is minus one below the norm and +1 is plus one above the norm, and so on.

Standard score (SS): another way to show where a student is placed in comparison to others of the same age. A standard score of 90 is the start of the average range, which is equal to a 25th percentile ranking. A standard score of 110 is the upper end of the average range and is equal to a percentile rank of 75.

Standardised test: a measure to judge a child's academic achievement in, for example, English reading, spelling or maths compared to other children throughout the country at the same class or age level

Stanford–Binet Intelligence Scales: a cognitive ability/IQ test that is used to diagnose developmental or intellectual deficits in children

STen Score: means a Score out of Ten; another way of comparing a child's performance against other children at the same age level

Suffix: a syllable placed at the end of a word that can further qualify the word such as indicating a tense, e.g. 'ing' or 'ed' in 'talking' or 'talked'

Syllable: the beat of a word; for example, 'car' has one syllable, while 'car-pet' has two

Syllable division rules: strategies that teach how to know where to split a word into its individual syllables or beats, demonstrating the rhythm of the word

Verbal comprehension: subsection of the WISC-IV cognitive test that measures a child's ability to understand, think and learn by using language and information already known, made by verbal instructions

Verbal instructions: giving oral/spoken instructions to be carried out

Glossary

Visual accommodation: being able to switch eye focus from long distance to short distance

Visual domain: visual area

Visual memory: an individual's ability to remember what has been seen

Visual motor integration difficulties: problems with integrating visual input with motor output, e.g. catching or hitting a ball

Visual perceptual difficulties: difficulties accurately perceiving what is seen; a sufferer may see blurred, moving or distorted images

Visualisation technique: a learning strategy using 'the mind's eye' to store and recall facts

Vocabulary repertoire: a person's range of vocabulary knowledge and understanding

Voice-activated technology: programs which 'write' what we wish to say and audio technology to 'read' aloud for us what we need to hear

Voice: the quality or tone of your voice when you speak

Vowels: the letters in the alphabet which are not consonants, i.e. A, E, I, O, U (and in my opinion 'Y'), which are made by vibrating the vocal cords without audible friction of the articulators (tongue, teeth or lips). Every syllable in the English language must have a vowel, but does not necessarily need a consonant.

Waiver: an allowance or dispensation that prevents an exam student from being penalised for spelling or grammatical errors in their written text

WIAT-II (Wechsler Individual Achievement Test – second edition): a test of ability in reading, spelling and maths

WISC-IV (Wechsler Intelligence Scale for Children – fourth edition UK): a cognitive assessment used by psychologists to measure the intellectual functioning of children from ages six to sixteen years

WordsWorthLearning programme: an online literacy programme for the remediation of reading and spelling difficulties in children and adults

Working memory: subsection of the WISC-IV cognitive test which measures short-term memory, i.e. the ability to take in, hold onto and reorganise lists of new information

Written language processing disorder: another term to describe difficulties experienced with understanding the written word, i.e. a reading comprehension difficulty